The Role of the
NVQ
Assessor

British Library Cataloguing in Publication Data

Day, Malcolm
    The role of the NVQ assessor: National Vocational
    Qualifications and the 'D' Units
    1. Nursing – Study and teaching – Great Britain – Evaluation
    2. Vocational education – Great Britain – Evaluation
    I. Title
    610.7'3'0711'41

ISBN 1 873732 23 6

©1996 Campion Press

Published by Campion Press
384 Lanark Road, Edinburgh EH13 0LX

Designed and typeset in 11/13pt Palatino
by Artisan Graphics, Edinburgh

Printed and bound by Bell and Bain, Glasgow

The Role of the
NVQ
Assessor

National Vocational Qualifications and the 'D' Units

MALCOLM DAY

M Ed, B Ed, RGN, RNT, Dip N (Lond) Cert Ed

City and Guilds Vocational Assessor and Internal Verifier (Awards)

Campion Press, Edinburgh

1996

Contents

About the author

Malcolm Day M Ed, B Ed, RGN, RNT, Dip N (Lond) Cert Ed, City and Guilds Vocational Assessor and Internal Verifier Awards.

Malcolm Day is a Senior Nursing Lecturer in the Department of Community and Primary Care of the School of Nursing and Midwifery at Sheffield University. He has had extensive teaching and management experience in pre- and post-registration nurse training, teacher and assessor staff development and continuing vocational education and training.

He was responsible for setting up the Sheffield and North Trent College and Employers' NVQ Consortium which was the first college-based consortium in the United Kingdom to be awarded a CCETSW kitemark of quality for vocational education and training.

As a Training and Development Consultant he assisted the Bromhead Hospital Consortium in Lincolnshire, the Edgefield and Glendaph Consortium in Herefordshire, the Goatacre Consortium in Wiltshire and the Old Rectory Nursing Home Consortium in South Yorkshire, to become approved NVQ centres.

He is Vice Chairman of the Health Care Tutors' Association, and has worked as an External Verifier for GNVQs in Health and Social Care.

Malcolm Day has been a regular contributor to *NVQ/SVQ Focus* and *Care Standard* magazines and has researched and written on issues relating to NVQ candidates' needs, the value of NVQs for Higher Education and the role and performance of NVQ assessors. He is a regular speaker on these issues at national and regional training and development conferences.

Introduction

This book is different! It is aimed at NVQ[1] assessors who state that their role can be significantly affected by:

- the use of complex jargon;
- the administrative requirements of assessment;
- conflicts between work and assessment roles;
- a lack of opportunity to practise.

To overcome these problems this book provides clear and explicit examples of what an assessor does, and how to make use of this as a basis towards achieving an NVQ Assessor Award.

Throughout the book, emphasis has been placed upon the personal experience of the assessor who is continually asked to review the implications NVQ requirements have on the practice of assessment in the workplace.

Although this book is primarily aimed at individuals working in the health care sector, care workers who are working in social care, child care, education, and the criminal justice field will also find parts of this book relevant and useful.

Nurse teachers in Schools of Nursing which have implemented competence-based approaches towards Project 2000 programmes will also find this book useful.

The contents of this book

Chapter 1 gives an account of the NVQ system and the implications this may have for the education and training of care workers, and for the practice of workplace assessment.

---

1 NVQs are National Vocational Qualifications, and SVQs are Scottish Vocational Qualifications. These are equivalent qualifications within the NCVQ framework, and while the book uses only the term NVQ throughout, the content applies equally to SVQs.

Chapter 2 outlines the role of the NVQ assessor and how it was determined by the Training and Development Lead Body. This chapter provides practical advice on choosing an appropriate Assessor Award, and how to register for this.

Chapter 3 provides practical advice to achieve the NVQ Assessor Award and examines what evidence qualifies towards this. This chapter includes advice on accreditation of prior learning and building a portfolio.

Chapter 4 examines the way in which assessors currently work, and the methods of assessment or evaluation they use. It also reviews factors which may inhibit the work of assessors and how these might be overcome.

Chapter 5 discusses study skills and provides further sources of information relating to each of the chapters outlined.

A Learning Record is provided in Appendix 2 to support the study activities in each chapter of the book.

How to use this book

For those who haven't registered for an Assessor Award, and who are new to the world of competence-based assessment, this book can be read chapter by chapter in order to gain an understanding of the role of the NVQ assessor and how to gain an Assessor Award.

Alternatively, those already registered to undertake an NVQ Assessor Award may wish to 'dip' in and out of relevant chapters to seek clarification or further help with:

– planning of assessment;
– maximising assessments;
– accreditation of prior learning;
– portfolio building;
– presenting a portfolio;
– study skills.

Study activities

Each chapter contains a series of study activities, with answers provided either in the text or the glossary. Further sources of information relating to these exercises, and how to access these sources, are given in Chapter 5.

Where study activities relate to the process of workplace assessment, assessor students should discuss the answers with their own assessor: this will enable them to generate evidence towards their NVQ Award. The Learning Record provided in Appendix 2 will help.

The following symbols are used throughout as prompts:

 Discuss with the assessor (or other person specified).

 Jot down your ideas and answers.

I hope you enjoy this book and wish you every success with your NVQ Assessor Award.

Malcolm Day

Spring 1996

CHAPTER ONE

National Vocational Qualifications

Introduction

This chapter outlines the development of the NVQ movement within the United Kingdom and the shaping of current NVQ in Care Awards. It takes a critical and uncompromising approach towards the question of workplace assessment and the factors which may influence this process. It will help with gaining a deeper understanding of the issues that may affect the development of the role of an assessor.

Learning outcomes

At the end of this chapter the assessor student will be able to:

1. trace the development of the Government's national occupational standards programme;
2. describe the NVQ framework and indicate its significance for the caring professions;
3. outline the role of Lead Bodies, Awarding Bodies and Accredited Centres;
4. outline the role and function of the NVQ Assessor, the Internal Verifier and External Verifier;
5. identify the factors which may influence the role and performance of an assessor.

National Vocational Qualifications

National Vocational Qualifications (NVQs) are endorsed by the National Council for Vocational Qualifications (NCVQ). These qualifications are based upon the skills, knowledge and understanding required for competence within a particular occupational area (NCVQ 1992 a). NVQs are concerned with outcomes rather than the learning process.

There are various ways of gaining an NVQ: following a formal training programme leading to an award; a mix of formal, informal or open learning approaches; or relying on past experience (NCVQ 1992 b).

NVQs are open to all, regardless of age, sex, race, special needs or prior qualifications (NCVQ 1992 c). Everyone has the opportunity to progress through a nationally recognised framework of qualifications which are based upon achieving competence no matter how it is acquired.

In order that a National Vocational Qualification can be accredited by the National Council for Vocational Qualifications, it must be based upon national standards for performance in employment. The award must also be free from any barriers restricting access and progression and be available to everyone able to reach the required standard, by whatever means.

National framework

All NVQs are accredited within a national framework according to progressive levels of achievement and areas of competence (NCVQ 1992 d). Refinements to the framework are made as qualifications are developed and routes for progression and transfer are identified. The function of the framework is to provide a coherent classification for NVQs, and to facilitate transfer and progression both within and between areas of competence.

The areas of competence defined in the framework are derived from an analysis of work roles, and they provide the organising structure for all competence-based qualifications within England, Wales and Northern Ireland. In Scotland these qualifications are known as Scottish Vocational Qualifications (SVQs) and are endorsed by the Scottish Council for Vocational Qualifications (SCOTVEC).

Currently the national framework defines 11 areas of occupational competence. Examples include construction, engineering and manufacturing. This book is concerned with NVQs in Care and the associated NVQs in Training and Development.

Levels, units, elements and performance criteria

NVQs are being developed to cover areas of competence at all levels, from the application of basic skills right through to professional understanding. For example, at the simplest level (Level 1) competence involves the

'... performance of work activities which are in the main routine and predictable or provide a broad foundation, primarily as a basis for "progression"'

      – National Council for Vocational Qualifications (1989), p10.

At the highest level (Level 5), on the other hand, competence

'... involves the application of a significant range of fundamental principles and complex techniques across a wide and often unpredictable variety of contexts. Very substantial personal autonomy and often significant responsibility for the work of others and for the allocation of substantial resources feature strongly, as do personal accountabilities for analysis and diagnosis, design, planning, execution and evaluation'

– Whitear (1993), p98.

Level 2 outcomes within the national framework are defined as

'... competence in a broader and more demanding range of work activities involving greater individual responsibility and autonomy than at Level 1'
– National Council for Vocational Qualifications (1989), p10.

Level 3 outcomes are defined as

'... competence in skilled areas that involve performance of a broad range of work activities, including many that are complex and non-routine. In some areas, supervisory competence may be a requirement at this level'
– National Council for Vocational Qualifications (1989), p10.

This book is concerned with NVQs in Care which are currently at Level 2 and 3, and with assessor qualifications which have been developed at Level 3 in training and development. At each level within the national framework, an NVQ is made up of several units of competence. A Unit is defined as the smallest grouping of performance standards that make up a key task or function within an occupational area (McCrory, 1992). Each unit of competence is made up of several elements (descriptions of employment expectations) and their associated performance criteria (the critical performances required in the workplace).

Lead and Awarding Bodies

Lead Bodies are employer-led organisations which represent the views of employers, trades unions and other interested parties within an employment area. Often working as Occupational Standards Councils, Lead Bodies are responsible for determining the standards required for satisfactory performance in employment.

Once the standards have been agreed, they form the basis for an NVQ which, subject to the criteria already discussed, is then endorsed by the National Council for Vocational Qualifications (NCVQ). The work of the Care Sector Consortium (Lead Body for care) and the Training and Development Lead Body is discussed throughout this book.

Lead Bodies are unable to award NVQs. This is the responsibility of the Awarding Bodies (for awards in care these are BTEC, City and Guilds and the Central Council for the Education and Training of Social Workers), who must be able to provide a programme matching the requirements of NCVQ and the Lead Body.

Once NCVQ has approved the performance standards agreed by the Lead Body and placed them within an area of competence and at a level within the national qualification framework, the Awarding Body may then offer the qualification to candidates through one of their accredited Assessment Centres.

Quality assurance

NCVQ is responsible for ensuring Awarding Bodies are adequately organised and resourced for quality assurance and that these systems operate effectively throughout the period for which the Awarding Body has received accreditation (Whitear, 1993). For example, NCVQ requires Awarding Bodies to have satisfactory dispositions to ensure the competence of assessors, to monitor the consistency and quality of evaluation, and to ensure adequate training and development of External Verifiers (moderators). In addition, Awarding Bodies must also allow external auditing of their NVQ programmes.

Awarding Bodies are responsible for verifying Assessment Centres have adequate arrangements and resources for quality assurance and that these systems operate effectively (Day, 1992; Waxman, 1993). These requirements are similar to those imposed by NCVQ upon the Awarding Bodies: they relate to the recruitment and development of candidates and the recruitment and development of assessors and Internal Verifiers (moderators). They also deal with the monitoring and evaluation of programme delivery and the communication and administration systems needed to support centre activities. The Assessment Centre is also required to participate in an audit which is carried out by an External Verifier appointed by the Awarding Body.

Central to the issue of quality assurance is the process of assessment or evaluation, in particular the degree to which the assessment is valid, reliable and sufficient (Jessup, 1991; Fletcher, 1991; McCrory, 1992). The recruitment, training and development of assessors have an important part to play in this process (Day, 1992, 1993; Mathias, 1993), a factor acknowledged by the publication of occupational standards for assessors (Training and Development Lead Body, 1992, 1995).

Study activity 1

Contact your local NVQ Co-ordinator and ask for a copy of the 1995

Training and Development Lead Body Standards. Look up the units and elements relating to the role of the assessor (D32 and D33), Internal Verifier (D34) and External Verifier (D35).

Now summarise in your own words the key functions of each of these individuals – it will be useful for you to look back at these summaries as you progress through this book. There is a difference between the elements constituting units D32 and D33. Can you explain this? Which elements are most appropriate to you?

You may also notice a difference between the elements of units D34 and D35. Can you account for this?

The glossary at the end of this book will help to clarify these points for you.

The United Kingdom and competence-based training

Concerns regarding the quality of vocational education and training programmes have been expressed by Government since the early 1980s. The New Training Initiative published by the Manpower Services Commission in 1981 was a forerunner to several major reports identifying the need for training to be closely relevant to the needs of industry to enable the United Kingdom to compete more effectively with other industrial nations. In this report the Manpower Services Commission called for the introduction of 'new standards' for training which would facilitate progress and adaptability within employment and improve access to training for young people and adults.

Although some of the recommendations of the Manpower Services Commission were introduced in the early 1980s, for example the Youth Training Scheme and the Technical Vocational Education Initiative, many political activists of the day argued that these schemes had been introduced with the sole aim of 'massaging' the rising unemployment statistics. Nevertheless, the idea that vocational education and training should meet the standards required for employment became a major driving force for education and training at the turn of the decade, one which many politicians, industrialists and trade unionists frequently referred to.

For example, in 1989 the Confederation of British Industry (CBI) reported that the skills of the United Kingdom workforce compared poorly with rival competitors, whilst the Trades Union Congress (TUC) Report of 1989 identified what it called the 'skills challenge' and stated a need to harness the potential of all workers by the year 2000, by which time the TUC suggested: '... *we will either be a superskills economy, or a low-skill, low-pay society'*.

In 1986 the Government undertook a review of vocational qualifications within the United Kingdom (Manpower Services Commission, 1986) and concluded there was no readily understandable pattern of provision, that duplication of qualifications by professional and industrial awarding bodies was evident, and that barriers to qualification arose from the attendance and entry requirements set by individual training programmes.

Further problems highlighted by the Manpower Services Commission (1986) included a lack of provision for progression and transfer of skills, both within and across occupational areas. Assessment within training programmes did not adequately test or record employment competencies and this was biased towards the recognition of knowledge and skills rather than occupational competence. As a consequence of this analysis, it was recommended that a new system of National Vocational Qualifications be set up, overseen by a National Council for Vocational Qualifications. This recommendation was implemented in October 1986.

The Training Agency of the Employment Department was established in 1988 in order to consolidate the work of the National Council for Vocational Qualifications. The Training Agency became responsible for working with employers, voluntary organisations, training providers and trade unions, in order to develop a United Kingdom-wide training system.

The Training Agency, briefed by the Employment Department, was to ensure that responsibility for training was accepted at a local level, that access to training throughout life be improved and that recognised standards of competence relevant to work would be established and recognised by industry.

In 1988 the Employment Department (now the Department for Education and Employment) published its national strategy for training. Based upon occupational standards for employment (determined by Lead Bodies), the Employment Department felt the emphasis should be upon the achievement of occupational competence.

Occupational standards and competence

Debling defined the concept of occupational competence as: '... *the ability to perform the activities within a function or an occupational area to the levels of performance expected in employment'.* – Debling (1989), p80.

Although this definition may appear paradoxical at times of rising unemployment, Debling argued that competence was a very broad concept which: '... *embodies the ability to transfer skills and knowledge to*

new situations within the occupational area. It encompasses organisation and planning of work, innovation and coping with non-routine activities.'
— Debling (1989), p80.

This broader notion of competence was highly relevant to a population whose working patterns were changing dramatically to include Government-sponsored community action programmes and voluntary work. Debling went on to indicate that a competent person could: *'... perform a particular function or role in a diversity of settings over a prolonged period of time and is able to respond to unique situations in differing environments.'* — Debling (1989), p80.

The need for people to be flexible and adaptable had become an essential characteristic as they might experience varied patterns of employment and several careers throughout their working life.

The responsibility for occupational standards development rested with Lead Bodies. Outcomes for an occupational area were determined by discussion, consultation and research. The principal method for standards development was through the process of functional analysis.

In this process experts from an occupational area identified the key purpose of that occupation by observing individuals going about their daily work. Analysis of these observations resulted in formulating a statement of what an employee had to do, and any qualifying factor (McCrory, 1992). Thus a statement of key purpose was written as follows:

DO   SOMETHING   TO AN AGREED STANDARD
(verb)   *(object)*   *(condition)*
— McCrory (1992), p25.

Figure 1.1 shows how each statement of key purpose (a unit) is further divided into elements (a description of the key activities

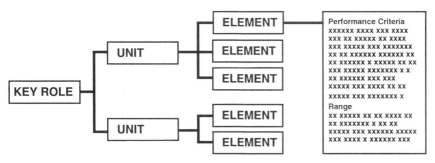

Figure 1.1 **The structure of standards**
(from Care Sector Consortium National Occupational Standards for Care, July 1992, piii)

19

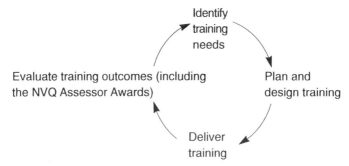

Figure 1.2 **The training cycle** *(Training and Development Lead Body, 1992)*

which make up a unit). Each element is further divided into the standards of performance required in order to successfully complete a key occupational role, or into performance criteria. For example, the key areas of training and development have been identified from a model of the training cycle (see Figure 1.2).

Each of the key areas relates to a stage in the training cycle. For example, look at the area of evaluation which is defined as: *'Area D: Evaluate the effectiveness of training and development.'* – Training and Development Lead Body (1992), p3. This has been further subdivided into:

Area D1 – Evaluate the effectiveness of training and development.

Area D2 – Evaluate individual and group achievement for public certification.

Area D3 – Assess achievement for public certification.

– Training and Development Lead Body (1992), p3.

The elements of Area D3 (*assess achievement for public certification*) include those activities that relate to the NVQ assessor's role, such as:

D321 – Identify opportunities for the collection of evidence of competent performance.

D322 – Collect and judge performance evidence against criteria.

– Training and Development Lead Body (1992), p16.

Once identified, occupational standards are developed by a further and wider process of consultation with employers (usually by postal survey). They are then field-tested within the appropriate occupational area and modified accordingly.

Criticisms of the NVQ approach

The development of occupational standards is a complex, systematic and carefully calculated process which aims to achieve high levels of validity and reliability through the conduct of consultation and field-testing (McCrory, 1992). However, there is some scepticism regarding the values and beliefs underlying the competence-based approach towards education and training. For example, in his critique of the NVQ movement, Robertson (1991) challenged the notion of *competence* which he considered dependent upon a poorly defined concept of learning.

Objections raised by Robertson (1991) included doubts about the origins and the worth of competence-based outcomes (or learning objectives) and doubts about the limitations of using linguistic statements to determine learning. With regard to the former, Professor Robertson questioned the degree to which competence-based outcomes truly reflected occupational (professional) values and judgements. With regard to his second reservation, Professor Robertson argued that linguistic learning outcomes were often ambiguous. Those which were unambiguous, he claimed, often trivialised the learning processes by their specificity. It was with this last point in mind that many educationalists criticised the role of functional analysis in determining occupational competence because it was regarded as being too prescriptive.

Elliot (1991) took up this argument and criticised what he saw as the development of a 'fundamentalist' approach towards education and training. Elliot claimed such a movement attempted to reduce social practices to a small number of essential elements, competence being regarded as an atomistic representation of a whole. In his critique of the NVQ movement Elliot described units and elements as having a unique and unquestionable (almost biblical) knowledge base. Thus he stated:

'As the Bible offers the assurance of salvation, so management science offers educational administrators an assurance of quality in an educational process conceived as a mode of production.'   – Elliot (1991), p120.

Elliot was concerned that the NVQ system had a potential to control and predict behaviour thereby devaluing the unique worth of an individual. Professor Robertson (1991) echoed this fear, suggesting that if NVQs were to have any credible influence upon the education system, they ought to be based upon the concept of 'excellence' rather than 'competence'.

Implications for education and training

The 'fundamentalist' approach towards occupational standards development has been criticised as being trivial, and of little worth. Such a response is characteristic of the debate between the value and purpose of *training* versus the value and purpose of *education*. For example, trainers often perceive education to be abstract, elitist and

Table 1.1
Training versus education
(adapted from Lawton, 1973)

Training	Education
Subject-centred	Student-centred
Skills	Creativity
Instruction	Experience
Information	Discovery
Obedience	Awareness
Conformity	Originality
Discipline	Freedom
Standards	Expression
Structure	Style
Unity	Diversity

socially divisive. Some educators on the other hand perceive training to be rather limited, mechanistic and at best a paradox (because training can no longer guarantee employment). These extreme and polarised views of the nature and purpose of education and training are compared and contrasted in Table 1.1.

However, distinctions between education and training are often unhelpful for they can be artificial and contrived – sometimes driven and reinforced by those who feel threatened and stand to lose status and power gained through academic credibility.

This is apparent within the Government's occupational standards programme which is largely controlled and delivered by institutions outside the mainstream of traditional education. Organisations such as local authority youth training schemes, in-service or in-company training departments, or private training companies have, for example, all enjoyed the support of Government funding in the implementation and delivery of NVQ programmes. This funding has allowed these organisations to grow and expand at a time when public sector funding for further and higher education has been severely restricted.

NVQs: education or training?

To demonstrate value and purpose, the outcomes of any programme of instruction must be clear and measurable. This is certainly the case with the unit-based performance criteria which make up an NVQ. With this in mind, the reader may be forgiven for thinking that NVQs could be classified as an example of the 'training' approach (see Table 1.1).

However, the principles of procedure inherent within the NVQ structure are drawn from philosophies reflecting a student-centred rather than a subject-centred model of education and training. For example, in their discussion paper 'Implications of competence-based curricula' in 1989, the Further Education Unit described what they considered to be a flexible and innovative response towards competence-based programmes (such as NVQs). This included:

- the development of training access points to improve access to educational information;
- the provision of a comprehensive counselling and profiling service;
- recognition of prior learning and experience;
- a modularised approach towards programme delivery;
- credit for individual modular achievements;
- a wider use of information technology to aid learning.

Greenacre (1990), in summarising the implications of changes within the post-compulsory curriculum, identified a need for:

- increased liaison with local industry (to include marketing and advisory services);
- increased communication with awarding bodies;
- the development of initial guidance and counselling services;
- the development of workshop, open learning and resource-based learning activities.

Greenacre went on to outline the importance of staff development within a college, identifying a need for *cross-curricula NVQ focus groups*. This has been recognised by the Further Education Unit (1989) who noted that further education colleges were now purchasers, rather than providers, of staff development, particularly when preparing staff for their new role in NVQ assessment. This cultural shift significantly altered the power base of teachers within the public education sector. They now became learners in association with their students – a feature Stenhouse (1975) perceived as representative of a student-centred curriculum.

This shift in power base, together with an emphasis on flexible and individualised programme delivery, is consistent with that advocated by Jessup (1991) in what he called 'the emerging model of education *and* training' (see Figure 1.3).

Study activity 2

What are your views on the NVQ debate?

In your opinion what are the strengths and weaknesses of the NVQ approach to education and training? Given your viewpoint, how might your opinions influence your work as an assessor? Will they cloud your judgement or influence your decisions in any way?

INFORMATION AND GUIDANCE
(career guidance, NVQ database, training access points,
educational counselling & credit transfer information service)

INITIAL ASSESSMENT
ACCREDITATION OF PRIOR LEARNING
(profiling of educational, workplace & non-workplace experiences)

INDIVIDUAL ACTION PLANS
(vocational and educational targets)

LEARNING OPPORTUNITIES
(workplace, college, open learning, resource-based learning)

CONTINUOUS ASSESSMENT
(varied locations, national records of achievement, unit accreditation)

NATIONAL VOCATIONAL QUALIFICATION
(achievement of action plan)

Figure 1.3 *The emerging model of education and training* (adapted from Jessup, 1991)

 Jot down your feelings; you will find it helpful to review these as you progress through this book.

Implications for the caring professions

In 1986 the United Kingdom Central Council for Nursing and Midwifery (UKCC) outlined a revised framework for professional nurse training. Known as 'Project 2000', the framework proposed major changes to training. They included the proposal that student nurses needed to have supernumerary rather than employee status, which would result in less student input into care delivery.

Although the recommendations of the United Kingdom Central Council (1986) were accepted by the profession, managers of care delivery had serious doubts about the manpower implications of removing what amounted to one third of the nursing workforce (the student nurses) from service provision. These doubts were echoed by the Government, who agreed to implement the 'Project 2000' recommendations provided that manpower issues could be addressed. In 1988, the Secretary of State for Health addressed the

Royal College of Nursing annual conference and outlined the Government's plan to introduce the 'support worker' to nursing and allied professions.

The job of introducing the support worker role was given to the National Health Service Training Directorate, who acted as secretary to the Care Sector Consortium (the Lead Body for care). The National Health Service Training Directorate were responsible to the National Health Service Management Executive, who were assigned the responsibility of implementing Department of Health policy, including the health care support worker role. Such an arrangement excluded direct influence from (or control by) the United Kingdom Central Council, the professional body for nurses (Davies, 1989).

The nursing profession's response to these arrangements was reactionary. The media carried headlines such as 'Nurse's little helper?', 'A special kind of person' (Dickson and Cole, 1987), and 'More of the same?' (Chudley, 1988). In 1987, an article by Hardie alluded to the need for support workers to have special nursing qualities in order that they may give patient care. Each of these expressed apprehension regarding the role of the support worker and its potential to 'de-skill' the process of care. They were also concerned that if the development of the support worker role was to retain a meaningful value, then it should be influenced by nurse education and the profession (National Federation for Educational Research, 1991).

Many professionals took a cynical view in outlining the reasons for the development of a support worker role. For example, Chapman (1990) highlighted Government strategy to limit National Health Service spending and suggested that by redefining the roles of people delivering care, the Government was able to demonstrate cost savings by creating a workforce which was cheaper to train and more flexible.

However, other professionals took a more pragmatic approach and recognised the need to determine workforce skills effectively in order that the quality of care delivery may be maintained. Storey (1991) argued that *'Support workers must be embraced as a supplement to nursing – not fended off as a threat to nursing…'*. In his analysis, Storey recognised that the prime reason for introducing the support worker role was an attempt to address the skills shortage brought about by reforms in nurse education.

Storey went on to indicate that NVQ training identified a unique role for the professional nurse in assessing support worker competence, thus ensuring that professionals had an opportunity to monitor and control the quality of care delivered by all members of the care team.

With this in mind, the Care Sector Consortium in 1990 set up the Health Care Support Worker Project which identified a qualification structure for health care support workers. And in 1992 the Consortium developed integrated occupational standards and a qualification structure for all health and social carers, whether they worked within the National Health Service, domiciliary, independent or voluntary sectors.

The integrated project (Care Sector Consortium, 1992) identified a qualification structure for those who '... *deliver hands-on care under the supervision, direction or guidance of qualified professional staff, such as nurses, midwives, health visitors, chiropodists, occupational therapists, physiotherapists, speech therapists and social workers ...*'

– Care Sector Consortium (1992), pi.

An outline of the qualification structure at Level 2 and 3 is given in Tables 1.2 and 1.3.

Core and value base units

NVQs in Care are based upon *Core Units* – key roles that all carers undertake (see Tables 1.2 and 1.3) – and a *core value base* or '*O*' *Unit*, which consist of elements relating to the care worker's role in:

– promoting anti-discriminatory practice;
– maintaining confidentiality;
– promoting and supporting individual rights and choice;
– acknowledging individuals' personal beliefs and identity;
– supporting individuals through effective communication.

The elements of the '*O*' *Unit* are continuously assessed throughout each unit of an NVQ in Care.

On achieving the *Core Units* a person is able to access an appropriate and relevant occupational or *Endorsement Unit*. Satisfactory completion of all Core Units and one Endorsement Unit leads to an NVQ award at Level 2 or 3.

The '*O*' *Unit* is a central focus for assessment across each of the units within a Level 2 or 3 award, thereby preventing fragmentation of what is essentially a modular curriculum. The elements and performance criteria within the '*O*' *Unit* address the issues that many authors such as Hardie (1987) raised when they questioned the purpose and value of the support worker in the caring relationship. It was also an attempt to define the attitudes or personal competencies unique to the care situation in order to reduce the possibility of purely mechanistic or skills-based behaviour.

The value of adopting occupational standards from NVQs in Care in

Table 1.2 **NVQs in Care: Level 2**
(adapted from Care Sector Consortium, 1992)

CORE UNITS (generic)	ENDORSEMENT UNITS (occupation specific)
'O' Unit: Promote equality for all individuals	Direct Care
Contribute to the protection of individuals from abuse	Developmental Care
	Domiciliary Support
Contribute to the ongoing support of clients and others significant to them	Residential/Hospital Support
Support clients in transition due to their care requirements	Post-Natal Care
	Special Care Needs
Contribute to the health, safety and security of individuals and their environment	
Obtain, transmit and store information relating to the delivery of a care service	

Table 1.3 **NVQs in Care: Level 3**
(adapted from Care Sector Consortium, 1992)

CORE UNITS (generic)	ENDORSEMENT UNITS (occupation specific)
'O' Unit: Promote Equality for all individuals	Promoting Independence
Contribute to the protection of individuals from abuse	Supported Living
	Rehabilitative Care
Contribute to the management of aggressive and abusive behaviour	Continuing Care
	Supportive long-term Care
Promote communication with clients where there are communication difficulties	Terminal Care
Support clients when they are distressed	Acute Care
Enable clients to make use of available services and information	Acute Care (children)
	Clinic and Out-Patient Care
Contribute to the health, safety and security of individuals and their environment	Substance Use
Obtain, transmit and store information relating to the delivery of a care service	Support and Protection
	Self-Environmental Management Skills
	Mental Health Care
	Mobility and Movement

order to complement the training of nurses and social workers has been recognised – particularly in applying the *'O' Unit* (Day and Basford, 1995; Storey et al., 1995).

Study activity 3

Obtain a copy of the occupational standards for care; your local NVQ Co-ordinator should have one.

Locate the elements that make up the *'O' Unit*. Consider these carefully and, in light of the exercises you have previously undertaken in this chapter, answer these questions:

1. How might you assess the *'O' Unit?*
   a) Through direct observation (D32).
   b) By collecting diverse evidence (D33).
   c) Both.

2. How trivial are the ideas and values expressed in the 'O' Unit? Given the underpinning values in this unit could you support the claim that NVQs are simplistic, and represent examples of relatively low levels of learning (Robertson, 1991)?

Jot down your ideas. You may want to return to these as you progress through the book.

Implications for workplace assessment

Jessup (1991) stated that evidence from NVQ assessment should be *valid, reliable* and *sufficient*. Thus:

Validity: the degree to which the assessment is based upon the competencies outlined in the appropriate units, elements and performance criteria. An assessment is said to be valid if the assessor refers only to these competencies.

Reliability: the consistency of assessment, the degree to which an assessor's opinion may match that of another assessor in the same situation, working with a similar candidate and applying the same occupational standards. Many Assessment Centres set up assessor panels which meet regularly to discuss consistency of approach towards assessment (Day, 1992).

Sufficiency: in order that an assessment may be judged sufficient, candidates must be able to demonstrate that all performance criteria and their corresponding range (specialised contextual and technical criteria) have been met. For example, the range for the Assessor Award includes evaluation of candidates who are confident as well as those who lack confidence, assessment of candidates within the workplace as well as candidates in the training environment.

Evaluation for an NVQ is a process of continuous assessment which may involve formative (diagnostic) as well as summative (terminal) assessment. Evidence submitted to substantiate a claim towards competence must also be

current: up to date;
authentic: the candidate's own work.

Assessment methods

NCVQ (1990) and the Joint Awarding Bodies (1992) saw the process of assessment as being criterion-led as well as candidate-centred. The candidate and assessor negotiated an appropriate plan of action for generating the evidence required to demonstrate competence. Much of this evidence originated in the workplace, the assessor observing the performance of the candidate and comparing this performance against the standards laid down.

Where performance evidence does not occur naturally, or in the case of evaluating underpinning knowledge and understanding, the assessor can question the candidate and make a judgement against the criteria set. Where assessment in the workplace is impossible for ethical or safety reasons, simulations, projects, assignments or skills tests can be used in conjunction with oral questioning.

Prior learning can also be recognised by adding direct evidence (examples of workplace products) or indirect evidence (employer testimonials) to a candidate's portfolio. Evidence of prior learning must meet validity, sufficiency, authenticity and currency requirements (Simosko, 1991, Royal Society of Arts, 1991).

The assessment methods for NVQs are summarised in Figure 1.4. They are discussed in greater detail in Chapter 3.

Potential problems

At first glance it may appear that the NVQ approach towards assessment offers a significant range of evaluation strategies in order to meet NCVQ's conditions of fairness, equal opportunity and quality.

However, there are potential flaws within the system. Some of the problems that could impinge upon and influence the outcomes of workplace assessment are: lack of familiarity with the occupational standard concerned, the occupational competence of the assessor, the terminology of occupational standards, the tedium and bureau-

UNITS, ELEMENTS AND PERFORMANCE CRITERIA
determine form and amount of evidence to be collected
using a combination of the following:

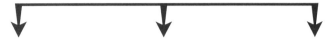

SUPPLEMENTARY EVIDENCE	EVIDENCE FROM PRIOR ACHIEVEMENT	PERFORMANCE EVIDENCE
gathered from:	*gathered from:*	*gathered from:*
oral questioning	reports, documents, products	observation in workplace
open written test	designs	extracted examples within workplace
structured written test	computer programmes	simulations
projects or assignments	testimonials from employers	skills tests
	certificates etc.	

*Figure 1.4 **NVQ assessment** (NCVQ, 1990)*

cracy associated with workplace assessment, and the occupational demands associated with the assessor's own job. For example, a training journal promoting a one-day training event called 'The Alphabet Soup!' printed:

'It's not that we don't agree with improving ourselves, other people and organisations! Who could argue with that? It's just that when we thought it was safe to go back in the water securely buoyant with our new-found knowledge and expertise about National Vocational Qualifications (NVQs), a whole ocean of acronyms suddenly appeared to potentially drown us again!' – NVQ/SVQ Focus (1993).

The title of this training event and its promotional hype may be amusing, but this coverage did reflect the climate of the vocational education and training culture which still found competence-based terminology difficult several years after the introduction of NVQs.

Further evidence by Mitchell (1993) suggested that broader principles relating to assessment of NVQs were narrowly and simplisticly interpreted by practitioners in the field:

'NCVQ and SCOTVEC focuses on a primary distinction between evidence of performance and evidence of knowledge and understanding (or that between direct and indirect evidence). However there are signs that this is not the interpretation which is received in the field. Evidence of performance is often interpreted as "evidence of performance which can be obtained via direct observation of activity"' – Mitchell (1993), p33.

Insisting that evidence could only be valid if it was directly observed through performance had manpower implications for many organisations. Such an approach also excluded indirect evidence like knowledge and understanding. Clearly there was a need to 'open up' assessment arrangements to make sure evaluations were valid, reliable and economic.

Further influences on the assessment process were identified by the Central Council for the Education and Training of Social Workers (1990) and the National Health Service Training Directorate (1991). These included:

The halo effect:	inferring competence on the basis of prior performance without attempting to validate this.
Stereotyping:	assuming competence on the basis of some apparent characteristic, e.g. once an assessor, always an assessor.
The contrast effect:	comparing the performance of a candidate with another, rather than with the occupational standards.
First impressions:	basing an opinion of the candidate as a result of the initial contact.
Similar-to-me:	judging candidates favourably because their performance mirrored that of the assessor.
Benefit of the doubt:	erring on the side of the candidate because most (rather than all) criteria had been met.
Experimenter effect:	if the candidate and assessor did not normally work together, the candidate could find the presence of the assessor intimidating.

In addition, Mullin (1992) identified the potential for 'false positive' outcomes in assessing NVQs, suggesting that the cause of this phenomenon may lie in the funding arrangements for NVQs, which are outcome driven. Therefore assessors may be under considerable pressure to 'pass' candidates and fulfil agreed training targets.

Implications for the role of the assessor

The introduction of achievement-led education and training has major implications for quality assurance, not least in the need to ensure adequate verification of assessment outcomes and in the development of those who undertake a key role in the evaluation process. This factor was recognised by the Joint Awarding Bodies (1992) who published guidelines for the selection and training of assessors for NVQs in Care.

For example, to become an assessor a person must be able to

demonstrate occupational competence in the areas they will be appraising, and familiarity with the principles of anti-discriminatory practice. They must also be able to demonstrate that they can work to the standards laid down by the Training and Development Lead Body.

However, these guidelines caused much confusion within health and social care organisations because there appeared to be a lack of consistency in their application. For example, the notion of 'adequate preparation' for the assessor's role has been questioned by Davies (1993) who noted that training could amount to as little as one day within some organisations. Davies went on to say: *'I would question the feasibility of such a programme and the fairness to both the assessor and his/her candidate and its contribution to the authenticity of NVQs.'*
– Davies (1993), p25.

In addition, the Joint Awarding Bodies require no proof (e.g. certification) of *occupational competence* for assessors, and although nurse practitioners must register with a professional body before being allowed to practise, this is not the case for those working in residential care – who may well be registered with the local authority, but have no professional qualification. This dual standard could call into doubt the validity of any assessment decision made by an assessor unable to demonstrate professional or occupational standards of competence. An example of this dual standard was experienced by the author who was asked to interpret occupational competence in care as: *'... being registered with the Local Authority as a carer'* – City and Guilds External Verifier for NVQs in Care, Lincolnshire (1993).

This begs the question as to whether all Local Authorities use the same criteria for registration or indeed have the same definition of the term *carer*. It is also in complete contrast to the interpretation by a different External Verifier within the South Yorkshire Region who stated that occupational competence was demonstrated by registration with a professional body.

 ## Study activity 4

With the help of the guidelines discussed in the chapter on study skills, search out and appraise the following article:

> Storey, L. (1995). Defining Occupational Competence for Assessors in Care. *NVQ/SVQ Focus and Care Standard.* Vol. 2, No. 12, pp. 36–37.

Now answer the following questions:

1. What are the key points raised in this article?
2. Do these key points present any difficulties for you?

3. If so, how will you resolve these?

You may wish to record your answers in the Learning Record (see Appendix 2).

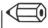

Equal opportunities and the assessor's role

With regard to requirements for anti-discriminatory practice the Joint Awarding Bodies indicate that assessors ought to tackle racism within the workplace by:

'confronting carers' racist assumptions about clients' needs, confronting assessors' assumptions about candidates from ethnic groups different from their own and helping to establish equal opportunities policies and statements.' – City and Guilds External Verifier Handout (1992).

These aims are laudable, but they contain negative assumptions and value judgements relating to professional care delivery over which the assessor may have little control and of which the External Verifier may have little knowledge. Furthermore, in highlighting these aims, the External Verifier may exacerbate existing stress by expecting the assessor to become an agent for change in addition to his or her role of assessor.

The Joint Awarding Bodies recognised the issue of role strain and role conflict for assessors by instituting guidelines for their recruitment, selection and training. They indicated that when establishing their role, potential assessors may expect some initial tensions within their organisations, including:

– tensions regarding the selection of one person as an assessor rather than another;
– tensions between assessor and manager when the assessor negotiates time and space out of normal work activities in order to carry out evaluations;
– personal tensions as assessors realise that they are held accountable for their evaluations;
– tensions when individuals realise the need to reconcile the demands of being an assessor with the demands of being a friend, colleague or supervisor.

Being an assessor entails dealing with various people both inside and outside an organisation (Joint Awarding Bodies, 1992). Associating with the NVQ candidate includes:

– pre-assessment guidance and action planning with candidates;
– observation and supervision of candidates;
– the provision of feedback on performance to candidates.

In addition, assessors are required to:

- meet with their peers for the purpose of standardisation of assessments;
- meet with External Verifiers to justify their evaluations;
- liaise between candidates and managers to report on candidate progress and to comment on resourcing.

Therefore the assessor's role is a highly complex one and, given the concerns already raised within this text, many are the factors which could impinge upon the performance of the assessor and upon the quality of the evaluation process.

Study activity 5

List the factors which may influence your role as an assessor. These could be reviewed under the following headings:

Your relationships with candidates.
Your relationships with peers.
Your relationships with managers.
Your workload.
Your competence as a professional carer.

You may wish to record your answers in the Learning Record (see Appendix 2).

Standards for NVQ assessment

The possibility of variation in assessment quality was recognised by the Training and Development Lead Body (1992, 1995) which developed occupational standards for assessors. Two major roles were recognised within these standards.

Firstly, standards relating to the role of the *first line* assessor. The first line assessor is defined as someone in a *front line* position within the workplace who will primarily appraise the candidate by direct observation of performance, supported by questioning to elicit underpinning knowledge and understanding. These standards comprise the following elements:

D32(1) – Agree and review a plan for assessing performance.
D32(2) – Collect and judge performance evidence against criteria.
D32(3) – Collect and judge knowledge evidence.
D32(4) – Make assessment decision and provide feedback.

Secondly, standards relating to the role of the *second line* assessor. The second line assessor is a person once-removed from the workplace who relies upon the judgement of peers and other assessors regarding candidates' performance. Thus the second line assessor relies upon a number of methods of evidence collection, as well as direct observation and the judgement of other assessors. These standards include the following:

D331 – Agree and review an assessment plan.
D332 – Judge evidence and provide feedback.
D333 – Make assessment decision using differing sources of evidence and provide feedback.

The term *peripatetic* has also been used by the Joint Awarding Bodies to describe the second line assessor role (Mathias, 1993). The Joint Awarding Bodies saw the peripatetic or itinerant assessor role as an opportunity to improve access for candidates who worked in isolated situations or without direct supervision, as do community workers or those working in child care, for example.

Study activity 6

Look back at the study activity in this chapter relating to the *'O' Unit*. Using the notes you made, consider the advantages of using:

1. direct observation;
2. diverse evidence.

Which do you think are the most valid and reliable means of assessing the requirements of the *'O' Unit*? You may wish to record your answers in the Learning Record (see Appendix 2).

The publication of standards for assessors is causing much controversy within the health care field, particularly as NCVQ, BTEC, City and Guilds and CCETSW are now seeking evidence that assessors meet TDLB standards before they can practise (Giles, 1993; NCVQ, 1993).

> ### Case study
>
> Many nurse practitioners with teaching and assessing qualifications gained through the English National Board 997/998 Teaching and Assessing in Clinical Practice course were surprised to learn that it does not meet the requirements of the Training and Development Lead Body and have reacted accordingly. For example, in a letter to the Joint Awarding Bodies, one assessment co-ordinator from a South Yorkshire Health Authority wrote:
>
> *'We are concerned that it is now deemed necessary for our already highly trained nurses and midwives to participate in another assessment programme. These members of staff have already been assessed in the skills of assessment, including teaching, giving*

Case study *continued*

feedback, evaluation, reflection, self-analysis, giving progress interviews, action planning etc.'
                                   – Letter to Senior Divisional Officer,
                                      City and Guilds, October 1992.

The letter went on to indicate the additional resourcing and costs involved in reassessing staff and the implications this would have on the workload of assessors and the morale of candidates. It continued:

'Are we to assume that the qualifications of those support workers who have already achieved Levels 1 and 2 are of less value because their assessors did not have the City and Guilds qualification in assessment?'

 Study activity 7

Consider the case history above. In light of the principles of NVQ assessment, how might you respond to the assessment co-ordinator? You might wish to consider the following points:

– the requirements of centre approval and the NCVQ common accord (1993);
– the experience of the 997/998 assessors and the context in which they have practised;
– the requirements of assessors to be familiar with the *'O' Unit*, and how this might be applied to the process of NVQ assessment.

For guidance, your local School of Nursing might provide an outline of the ENB 997/998 Teaching and Assessing in Clinical Practice syllabus. Alternatively, you may contact the English National Board for Nursing, Midwifery and Health Visiting (telephone 0171 388 3131). You may wish to record your answers in the Learning Record (see Appendix 2).

Summary

This chapter has attempted to identify the political, economic and educational influences behind the organisation and development of NVQs within the United Kingdom, and the influence this has had upon the education system, workplace assessment, nursing and other care professions.

A critical approach has been undertaken in order that the relative strengths and weaknesses of the NVQ system may be appreciated.

Such an approach will help the assessor student to develop a greater awareness of the underlying principles of NVQ assessment and the factors which may influence this.

End of chapter activity

It may be helpful for you to review the following key points. You can check your answers in the Glossary at the end of the book.

1. Describe what is meant by a *unit*.
2. Describe what is meant by an *element*.
3. What are *Performance Criteria*?
4. What is an *Endorsement Unit*?
5. What are *Core Units*?
6. What is the *'O' Unit*?
7. What are the key roles of the *first line assessor* (D32)?
8. What are the key roles of the *second line assessor* (D33)?
9. What are the key roles of the *Internal Verifier* (D34)?
10. What are the key roles of the *External Verifier* (D35)?
11. What are *Lead Bodies*?

You may wish to record your answers in the Learning Record (see Appendix 2).

CHAPTER TWO

Occupational standards for NVQ assessors

Introduction

The last chapter examined in some detail the NVQ system within the United Kingdom and the political and educational factors to influence its development. As seen, the potential for bias and misinterpretation during the process of evaluation at work is great.

However, NCVQ and SCOTVEC have attempted to address this by:

– specifying assessment outcomes in the form of national occupational standards;
– introducing a national accreditation and verification system;
– developing guidelines and criteria for approval of NVQ Assessment Centres;
– introducing standards for assessors and verifiers.

This chapter will look in more detail at the national occupational standards for NVQ assessors and how these determine the assessor role and function.

```
┌─── Learning outcomes ──────────────────────
│ At the end of this chapter the assessor student will be
│ able to:
│ 1. outline the role of the 'first' and 'second line'
│    assessors;
│ 2. describe the role of the assessor in planning for
│    assessments;
│ 3. describe the role of the assessor in collecting
│    evidence;
│ 4. describe the role of the assessor in giving feedback
│    to candidates;
│ 5. register for an appropriate NVQ Assessor Award.
└────────────────────────────────────────────
```

The first line assessor

It was shown in Chapter 1 that national occupational standards for first line assessors are outlined within TDLB unit D32 (Training and Development Lead Body 1992, 1995). The elements of unit D32 include:

D32(1) – Agree and review a plan for assessing performance.
D32(2) – Collect and judge performance evidence against
        criteria.
D32(3) – Collect and judge knowledge evidence.
D32(4) – Make assessment decision and feedback.

D32(1) Agree and review a plan for assessing performance

This unit demands assessors to plan the most appropriate time, place and evaluation method with their candidate. There is no prescribed format for this but the following will need to be taken into account and discussed with the candidate:

- the unit and performance criteria to be examined;
- an appropriate time and place for the assessment;
- the type of evidence the assessor will be gathering, i.e. how to judge performance as well as the underpinning knowledge;
- any aspects of confidentiality that may apply to clients or patients;
- any ethical implications, e.g. will the patient or client agree to participate in the assessment? How will the safety of any third party be maintained?
- any special requirements – the candidate might be a night worker, be nervous, have impaired hearing or speak English as a second language;
- finally, assessor and candidate will need to make sure that all parties to the assessment agree with the intended plan of action and that this agreement is recorded on an assessment plan (see Figure 2.1).

D32(2) Collect and judge performance evidence against criteria

The assessor judges a candidate's performance of a particular task against the performance criteria for the unit appraised. The performance criteria are to be found in the candidate's Record of Assessment: these should be available when assessing the candidate. It will also be useful to draw up a checklist to refer to (see Figure 2.2).

The candidate will be observed whilst undertaking tasks and activities at work, spontaneous or planned. This evaluation method can be difficult to support without checklists, which should be signed by the candidate and assessor.

Assessment plan

Candidate's name: Awarding Body No.:
Centre name: Assessor:
Unit(s): Z6, Z9 and Z10   Element(s): All

1. Assessment opportunities:
Candidate to work with a group of five heavily dependent and immobile
patients recovering from the effects of a stroke. Care activities undertaken
by the candidate to include assistance with personal hygiene, eating and
drinking and mobility needs.

2. Assessment methods:
Direct observation of care activities during a span of duty to be followed by
a question and answer discussion to draw out *range* and *underpinning
knowledge.*

Presentation of copy care plans in candidate's portfolio to show entries
made by candidate relating to the assessment and care given to each
patient (where appropriate).

3. Resources required:
Performance criteria and assessment requirements for Units Z6, Z9 and
Z10
Care plans
Candidate's portfolio of evidence
Candidate's record of assessment

4. Action to be taken by assessor:
To act as assistant to candidate. To intervene only in the case of unsafe
practice or in the event of an emergency.

5. Action to be taken by candidate:
Seek patient's permission for the assessment to take place.
Assess and plan patient's needs for the span of duty and confirm these
with the *named nurse.*
Complete sections of the care plan which cover assessment and
intervention for each of the five patients.
Submit a copy of each of these care plan entries in the portfolio of
evidence.
Submit record of assessment and portfolio to the assessor on the
completion date agreed.

6. Signed (candidate):   Date:

   Signed (assessor):   Date:

*Figure 2.1 **An assessment plan***

Assessment checklist

Candidate's name: Awarding Body no.:
Centre name: Assessor:
Unit(s):   Element(s):   Date:

Performance criteria	Assessor comments
1	
2	
3	
4	
5	
6	
7	
8	
9	
10	
11	
12	

Evidence for *range:*

Evidence of *underpinning knowledge:*

Signed (candidate):   Date:

Signed (assessor):   Date:

Figure 2.2 **Assessment checklist**

To help validate assessment decisions it is often helpful to refer to, and collect examples of 'products' that have arisen from the candidate's work during the observation period, such as copies of care plans, fluid charts, temperature charts etc. These should be relevant to the performance criteria examined, and should also provide evidence to meet the range requirements.

D32(3) Collect and judge knowledge evidence

This is concerned with asking the candidate questions to support the observations made of their performance. The questions should cover the range requirements and underpinning knowledge relating to the element assessed. It is important not to 'lead' the candidate, i.e. the question must not suggest the answer.

Questions could be asked during the period of observation, or they could be asked at the end of the observed activity. They may be:

spontaneous – oral questions arising naturally from the observations made. It is advisable to jot these down as well as the candidate's response, as far as is reasonably possible (i.e. this should not be allowed to distract from the observations);

pre-planned – a series of written questions asked at the end of the observation period. In fact, together with colleagues, the assessor could develop a 'question bank' for use with candidates. The advantage is that other assessors can cross-validate the questions and ascertain they directly relate to the element concerned. It is important that these questions should not be divulged to candidates prior to their assessment;

or *both* – growing familiarity with the requirements of the standards and more experience in the art of questioning will engender the wish to combine both strategies in order to gain a greater appreciation of the candidate's performance and underpinning knowledge. The questions should cover the processes observed as well as the outcomes. It is important to pay particular attention to the range requirements (i.e. questions about the contexts and situations which it was not possible to observe).

Candidates can become nervous when subjected to questioning. It is not uncommon for a complex question put during the observation period to go unanswered: the candidate is probably too busy caring for the client! In this situation questions are best kept simple and should relate directly to the performance (or process) observed.

If questioning takes place at the end of the observation period, a quiet room is needed, free from interruptions and distractions. This could be done over a cup of coffee, for example. It is helpful to list the questions on a separate sheet of paper to refer to. This sheet should also have a blank column in which to record the candidate's answers. Both the assessor and the candidate will then sign it.

Some guidelines on how to ask questions are provided in Table 2.1.

D32(4) Make assessment decision and feedback

Once all the evidence needed to decide whether a candidate meets

43

Table 2.1 **The art of questioning**

ASKING QUESTIONS

A candidate has to hear, understand, think about, search their memory, formulate an answer and then give an answer to any question asked. This all takes time.

Do:	Don't:
Ask questions in an interested manner and in a natural tone of voice.	Say 'Are you sure?' (in any tone of voice) after any answer that is correct.
Put the questions in plain, simple language, avoiding jargon.	Be sarcastic at wrong answers.
Give the candidate time before moving on to the next question.	Ask trick questions.
Ask questions which require more than a one-word Yes/No answer.	Intimidate the candidate.
	Ask mainly factual questions.
Phrase the questions so that they do not lead the candidate, i.e. the question does not suggest the answer.	Repeat the question (it is probably better to rephrase it).
Make sure the questions are not ambiguous.	Ask questions 'for the sake of asking'.
Always encourage a full answer.	
Give praise and encouragement for any correct answers received.	

The questions asked must be valid, i.e. directly related to the requirements of the element and performance criteria examined.

the required standard has been collected, the candidate has to be informed. It is good to give praise where it's due – to say that the candidate is 'competent' is a poor substitute for praising excellence, when it occurs!

Similarly, if the standards outlined within the performance criteria or the range have not been met, the candidate has to be told in a positive and constructive manner how the shortfall can be made up.

This has to be done in a clear and concise fashion – in fact, it would be helpful to record this information for the candidate (a sample record is provided in Figure 2.3).

The candidate will be anxious. Any comment can be potentially destructive: the assessor needs to call on good powers of communication to handle this situation as sensitively as possible.

A way of doing this could be to ask candidates how they thought they had got on. This will 'open up' the feedback process, and allow the

Record of feedback and advice given

NVQ in Care candidate's name:

Assessed for level: Unit: Element(s):

Evidence methods used:

Areas where competence achieved:

Areas where competence has not yet been achieved:

Assessor's comments:

Candidate's comments:

Signed (assessor student):   Date:

Signed (NVQ in Care candidate):   Date:

Figure 2.3 **Record of feedback and advice given**

candidate to identify weaknesses without fear of external criticism. As a result, the candidate will often identify the shortfall observed, leaving the assessor to build upon the candidate's strong points, and reassure them that the shortfall can be overcome.

Setting time aside and having a quiet room free from interruptions will help. However, it is the assessor's personal approach and the way in which interest and concern are conveyed that will ensure a successful outcome to this process. Here are some guidelines:

First,
- ensure the room has enough seating and space for you and your candidate;
- remove any physical barriers, such as desks or tables – sit alongside your candidate;
- smile, ask if the candidate is comfortable, and whether he or she would like a refreshment;
- don't crowd your candidate – allow them room to breathe!
- convey interest by maintaining steady eye contact – don't stare, though!
- be aware of your posture and body language – folded arms or 'finger pointing' can be quite threatening.

Then,
- explain the purpose of the meeting;
- ask the candidate how they thought they got on – don't allow them to be too negative!
- add any comments you have to complement your candidate's observations;
- highlight the candidate's strengths – praise these;
- highlight shortfalls – maintain your objectivity by referring to the criteria for assessment;
- encourage your candidate to ask questions, and to put their point of view;
- record the outcomes of the discussion, making sure you and your candidate each have a copy;
- finally, thank your candidate for participating in the discussion.

The second line assessor

Chapter 1 described how national occupational standards for the second line assessor were outlined within TDLB unit D33: *Assess candidate using differing sources of evidence.* The elements of unit D33 include:

D33(1) – agree and review an assessment plan;
D33(2) – judge evidence and provide feedback;
D33(3) – make assessment decision using differing sources of

evidence and provide feedback.

The stages of the NVQ assessment process associated with these elements are similar to those previously outlined, that is:

– planning for the assessment;
– collecting evidence;
– making a judgement;
– giving feedback.

However, a second line assessor is 'once-removed' from the workplace and will not always directly observe the candidate whilst at work. Thus, in addition to direct observation and questioning, the second line assessor will also be drawing upon other methods of evaluation to make a final judgement of the candidate's competence. These methods might include:

– reports from the candidate;
– reports from the candidate's peers;
– testimonials;
– simulation;
– recognition of prior achievements and learning.

In this situation the process of assessment will include:

– planning for the assessment;
– collecting evidence;
– making an initial judgement and giving feedback to the candidate;
– making a final decision based upon other evidence received.

Each of the possible assessment methods, and how they may relate to the achievement of the NVQ Assessor Award are discussed in the next chapter.

Summary

This chapter looked in detail at the national occupational standards for NVQ assessors and at the way in which the assessor's role and function are determined by these.

In particular, it examined the activities undertaken by 'first line' and 'second line' assessors, and highlighted the different assessment methods they used.

Study activity 8

This activity prompts you to examine your role as an NVQ assessor to help you decide which NVQ Assessor Award you should register for.

Look back at the study activity you undertook in Chapter 1. This identified the differences between 'first line' and 'second line' assessors. Which do you think is the most appropriate for you? Will you be working directly alongside your candidate and observing their performance during the normal course of their work? Or do you have more of a supervisory role, relying on others to testify on your candidate's performance, or relying on evaluation methods other than direct observation of your candidate?

Perhaps you want to develop competencies from units D32 *and* D33, in order to carry out direct observation and exercise various methods of assessment. This is particularly important if you are:

– a supervisor of night workers: here opportunities to directly observe are often reduced;
– a peripatetic assessor: surveying candidates within and across many different organisations; or
– working in an area where informed consent and client confidentiality are of *primary* importance.

Your decision will be dependent upon the type of organisation you work for and your role within it, and also upon whether your NVQ programme is delivered in-house or by an external centre. Your manager or your NVQ Co-ordinator will be of help here.

Whatever your decision, be honest about your responsibilities as an assessor. You will not be able to achieve your Assessor Award unless you meet all of the elements, performance criteria *and* range statements of the appropriate 'D' Units.

End of chapter activity

By now you will have a pretty good idea of which TDLB award(s) you want to gain. However, before you register with an Accredited Centre, it is worth spending time to consider what your assessment and training needs might be.

Using the guidelines discussed in the chapter on study skills, search out and appraise the following article:

Pitchford, S. (1995). Choosing the right centre for your company training and development awards. *NVQ/SVQ Focus and Care Standard*. Vol. 2, No. 12, pp6,7.

Now answer the following questions:

1. What are the key points raised in this article?
2. Do these key points raise any issues for you as an assessor student?
3. If so, how will you resolve these?

CHAPTER THREE

Collecting evidence for units D32 and D33

Introduction

The aim of the last chapter was to provide a detailed analysis of the role of the NVQ assessor to help decide which Assessor Award to undertake, and to provide guidance in helping to register for this.

This chapter will concentrate on issues relating to the collection of evidence. In particular, it will review what is meant by *sufficient evidence* in relation to:

− direct observation of performance;
− use of candidate and peer reports;
− assessment records;
− use of simulations.

It will also provide guidance on *recognition of prior learning and achievement* and the *development of portfolios*.

Examples relating to the assessment requirements for unit D32 and D33 are given to help clarify what is acceptable evidence towards an NVQ Assessor's Award.

Learning outcomes

At the end of this chapter the assessor student will be able to:

1. describe what is meant by *sufficiency* of evidence;
2. discuss the use of observation of performance as an evaluation method;
3. discuss the use of candidate and peer reports, testimony of others and simulation;
4. describe the requirements for recognition of prior learning and achievement;
5. discuss the implications for developing a portfolio of evidence.

Principles of NVQ assessment

Whatever methods are chosen to appraise candidates, the fundamental principles remain the same. These include the need to ensure the following:

Validity – assessments should be based upon the standards outlined in the appropriate units, elements and performance criteria – in the case of assessor students these relate to units D32 and/or D33.

Reliability – is the performance of the assessor student *consistent*? If evaluated in the same way, against the same standards, but on different occasions, will the performance of the assessor student be the same?

Sufficiency – assessor students must be able to demonstrate that all performance criteria, their range and underpinning knowledge have been met.

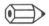

Study activity 9

Using the guidelines in the chapter on study skills, search out and appraise the following articles:

> Raggat, P. and Hevey, D. (1995). Do I have enough Evidence? *Competence and Assessment*. Employment Department. Issue 27, pp10–12. Sheffield.

> Heaton, M. (1995). Standardisation: What is enough evidence? *Association for Social Care Training*. Conference Newsletter. July 1995, p24.

Now answer the following questions:

1. What are the key points raised in this article?
2. Do these key points raise any issues for you as an assessor student?
3. If so, how will you resolve these?

You may wish to record your answers in the Learning Record (see Appendix 2).

Assessment by direct observation

Much of the evidence produced towards an NVQ Assessor Award will arise as a result of being observed. At the end of the observation period the assessor may wish to question the assessor student on some aspect of their performance in order to check underpinning knowledge, or to ensure that the range requirements of the unit have been met.

For example, the range requirements for D32 demand that assessor students show they have observed both *processes* and *products* arising from the work situation, i.e. the process of giving care as well as the result, or outcome.

They also need to demonstrate they are able to work with experienced and inexperienced candidates, confident and less confident candidates, as well as those with special assessment requirements.

Assessor students must be able to display a range of questioning methods, such as written and oral questions, spontaneous and preset questions. Many of these range requirements were discussed in Chapter 2. At the end of this question and answer session, the assessor will discuss the assessor student's performance and together they will record what happened. This record is made on the evidence log, which can be found in the Record of Assessment given after registering for the Assessor Award.

Evidence log

Evidence logs vary according to awarding body stipulations, but generally they require:

- the date the assessment took place;
- the method of assessment;
- description of the assessment;
- cross-reference of the assessment activity to the performance criteria concerned.

The assessor student and the assessor then sign and date the log. The number of entries in the evidence log increases until the assessor pronounces the student as competent. At this point they both sign the Record of Assessment, carefully indicating the units for which competence has been reached.

Using different assessment methods

It may be that evidence of the 'range' or 'underpinning knowledge' does not naturally emerge from the assessment being observed. In this case, as well as answering the assessor's questions the assessor student may wish to put forward other evidence to support a claim to competence. Such evidence might include a report from:

- the assessor student (on other assessments already undertaken – see Figure 3.1);
- the NVQ candidate (on how the assessor student conducted any previous assessments – see Figure 3.2).

It may also include a record of any learning gathered whilst practising as an assessor to supply evidence of underpinning knowledge. For example, the Learning Record which is provided in Appendix 2

Assessor student's report

NVQ in Care candidate's name:

Assessor student's name:

NVQ candidate is registered for:

State which unit is being assessed:

State which element is being assessed:

Briefly outline the assessment activity:

State how the performance criteria have been met:

performance criteria	explanation
a	
b	
c	
d	
e	
f	
g	

Signed (assessor student):   Date:

Signed (NVQ in Care candidate):   Date:

Figure 3.1 (above) **Assessor student report on assessment activities undertaken**

Figure 3.2 (opposite) **A carer's report on assessment activities undertaken by an assessor student**

NVQ in Care candidate's report

NVQ in Care candidate's name:

Assessor student's name:

NVQ in Care candidate is registered for:

State which unit is being assessed:

State which element is being assessed:

Briefly outline the assessment activity:

Did the assessor student:	Comments
Give clear information relating to your assessment?	
Encourage you to identify and present relevant evidence?	
Involve you in planning your assessment?	
Only assess you against the performance criteria?	
Use clear and concise questions?	
Use justifiable questions?	
Confirm success when evidence was sufficient?	
Give feedback as soon as practicable?	
Give clear and concise feedback?	
Give constructive feedback?	
Encourage you to put your point of view?	
Encourage you to ask questions?	
Record the outcomes of your assessment whilst you were present?	

Signed (NVQ in Care candidate):   Date:

Signed (assessor student):   Date:

could be used to record the answers to the various study activities in this book.

Testimonials

In addition to the assessor student's or the NVQ candidate's reports, a supervisor with personal knowledge of the assessor student's work might write a testimonial. Each example of work needs to be cross-referenced to an appropriate performance criterion, and the author of the testimonial has to be competent in the area commented on. Presentation of the testimonial on letter-headed paper, dated, signed and with the writer's professional qualifications after the signature, will help to validate the document.

Study activity 10

With the help of the guidelines in the chapter on study skills, search out and appraise the following article:

Novik, T. (1995). 'She's usually very helpful ...' Using the testimony of others. *The Association of Social Care Trainers*. September 1995 Newsletter, p7.

Now answer the following questions:

1. What are the key points raised in this article?
2. Do these key points raise any issues for you?
3. If so, how will you resolve these?

You may wish to record your answers in the Learning Record (see Appendix 2).

Assessment records

Alternatively, assessor students might choose to provide examples of assessment plans and records they have written or completed. Provided the confidentiality of the NVQ candidate and their client is maintained, these records or 'products' are acceptable evidence towards the Assessor Award. These could be copies of the candidate's record of assessment and their evidence logs, together with a copy of the standards covered.

Simulation

The use of simulation is an acceptable means of generating evidence towards an NVQ. It may also be of value as a training exercise, e.g. in learning how to construct an assessment plan or to give feedback to a candidate.

Simulation may be used when assessing an NVQ in Care candidate – for example, when judging a candidate's response to fire or to cardiac arrest. However, using simulation as a means of generating evidence towards the NVQ Assessor Award has limitations.

The next study activity looks at these issues. The answers can be recorded in the Learning Record provided in Appendix 2, and submitted as evidence towards the Assessor Award.

Study activity 11

With the help of the guidelines in the chapter on study skills, search out and appraise the following article:

Mansfield, B. (1995). Simulation – A necessary evil or acceptable source of evidence. *The NVQ Monitor.* Summer 1995, pp3–6.

Now answer the following questions:

1. What are the key points raised in this article?
2. Do these key points raise any issues for you?
3. If so, how will you resolve these?

You may wish to record your answers in the Learning Record (see Appendix 2).

There are endless opportunities to generate evidence towards an Assessor Award. At first the idea of generating evidence might appear daunting, but it is not difficult to see how evidence emerges naturally from the daily activities undertaken in the role of assessor.

Assessor students may feel they already have the necessary knowledge and experience required to meet some or all of the performance criteria of the units relating to their Assessor Award. If so, they should ask their assessor about accreditation of prior achievements.

Accreditation of prior achievement

Evidence of prior learning and achievement is another form of acceptable evidence. Much of the allowable evidence has already been discussed, and includes:

1. certificates from previous courses, e.g. ENB 997/998, City and Guilds 730 award etc.;
2. records of learning (see Appendix 2);
3. work records;
4. assessment records;
5. candidate reports;
6. testimony from others.

Experienced trainers or supervisors may feel they already have evidence from prior achievements. Some organisations, for example, keep a comprehensive account of staff training and may also carry out regular staff performance and review interviews. Other organisations issue workers with a personal handbook to record supervisors' comments on work performance. The outcomes of these staff development activities can be used as evidence, provided they relate to the performance criteria of the Assessor Award, and provided they can be substantiated.

It is worth thinking about the evidence already accumulated. For example, consider the element D32(1) *agree and review a plan for assessing performance.*

This element is an important part of a supervisor's or trainer's role. It is therefore likely that the assessor student will have accumulated some evidence to demonstrate competence in these activities, particularly in the process of planning and organising evaluations against specific criteria.

Each of these pieces of evidence can be accumulated and presented in a personal profile to the assessor for consideration against the appropriate element and performance criteria.

Study activity 12: reviewing prior achievements

Take your record of assessment and locate unit D32. Consider each of the 4 elements and their performance criteria. Now build up a profile of competence using the grid in Figure 3.4.

For example, if you have an ENB 997/998 Certificate, a City and Guilds 929 Award, or a Teaching Certificate such as the City and Guilds 730, you will almost certainly have some evidence towards D323 *collect and judge knowledge evidence*, particularly on the use of oral or written questioning. So write c, d, e and f in the *performance*

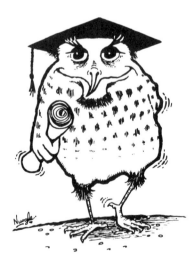

Figure 3.3 **The wise owl: assessor students may feel they already have the necessary knowledge.**

criteria column on the left, then tick columns 1, 3 and 5 on the right to show how you support your claim to competence, and so on, until you have built a profile of your competencies relating to unit D32.

When you have completed your profile, discuss it with your assessor. Don't be surprised if your assessor questions what you have written; this is part of the evaluation process and you both need to be sure that the evidence presented meets the requirements of the Awarding Body. This is particularly important to meet *range* and *underpinning knowledge* requirements.

At the end of this exercise you will have built up a personal profile to support your claim to competence in unit D32, which you can place in your portfolio. You will also have identified any areas where

---

Assessment grid for accrediting prior achievement

Candidate's name: Awarding Body no.:
Centre name: Assessor:
Unit(s):   Element(s):   Date:

Performance Criteria   Types of Evidence
                                           (see key below)

	1	2	3	4	5
a					
b					
c					
d					
e					
f					
g					

Evidence Key   1. Certificates from previous courses.
                2. Records of learning (see Appendix 2).
                3. Assessment records.
                4. Candidate reports.
                5. Testimony from others.

Evidence for range:

Evidence of underpinning knowledge:

Signed (candidate):   Date:

Signed (assessor):   Date:

*Figure 3.4 **Assessment grid for accrediting prior achievement***

further guidance and support are needed, e.g. in the range requirements of unit D32. If you wish, you could repeat this exercise with unit D33.

Organising and planning assessments

As well as identifying evidence of prior achievement it may be possible to organise work so that it can be examined against several units and elements at the same time. For example, unit D32 encompasses the process of action planning and giving feedback and these activities also relate to unit D33 (see Chapter 2).

To be meaningful, it is recommended to use a *whole* or *holistic* approach towards assessment, rather than reduce the process to a series of unconnected observations and tasks.

Benefits of care in organisation and planning

It is well worth carefully planning assessments in order to:

1. make them more interesting;
2. make them more meaningful;
3. prevent unnecessary repetition;
4. maximise achievements;
5. save valuable time, which can then be applied elsewhere.

As well as taking great care over planning the assessments, it will also be necessary to take care over how work (and learning) is organised so as to make the best use of the evidence generated. One way of doing this is to build up a *portfolio* of work.

The portfolio

A portfolio is a record of work experience and personal development

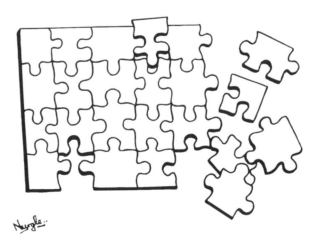

*Figure 3.5 **Holistic approach to assessment***

built up over time in order to support a claim to competence. It is a folder or file which contains:

1. the student assessor's plans for training and assessment;
2. a review of actions since starting the Assessor Award;
3. descriptions of the activities undertaken at work;
4. evidence from colleagues and others about the student assessor's skills and abilities.

A portfolio provides a way to give a comprehensive account of skills and abilities in relation to the NVQ Award undertaken. To do this it should:

- be structured clearly and logically;
- be supported by evidence from colleagues and other health care professionals;
- describe the student's role as an assessor and the work environment;
- be easy to read and understand;
- allow some freedom of expression.

Presenting a portfolio

The presentation of the portfolio is crucial. It should be easy to follow and the assessor should readily be able to identify the evidence that supports claims to competence in each unit.

There should be a contents page outlining each section of the portfolio – a spare evidence log could serve for this. Each section should represent one unit, and should contain the evidence collected – this must be complete, signed, dated and appropriately cross-referenced to the evidence log. (Cross-referencing could be done numerically or with colour codes.)

Each section should then be prefaced by a brief summary of its content, rather like the introduction to this book.

The assessor may reject the portfolio if it is poorly presented, so it is important to make sure the assessor student's name is clearly printed throughout the reports, that documents and records are legible, and the portfolio is neatly bound and assembled.

Learning how to develop a portfolio

One of the most difficult tasks in compiling a portfolio is deciding what to include. The possible sources of evidence for an NVQ have already been discussed. However, the art of building a portfolio is a learning process in itself and includes the following stages:

1. familiarisation with the standards and the NVQ framework;

2. a review of existing abilities and prior achievements;
3. self-assessment and production of a personal profile;
4. identifying personal development needs;
5. identifying other sources of help and guidance;
6. identifying appropriate sources of evidence;
7. identifying opportunities to maximise evidence generation;
8. planning and organising assessments towards NVQ Assessor Award;
9. compiling the evidence.

Study activity 13

With the help of the guidelines in the chapter on study skills, search out and appraise the following article:

Lavelle, J. (1995). Jurassic Portfolio? *NVQ/SVQ Focus and Care Standard.* Vol. 2, No. 12, pp22–25.

Now answer the following questions:

1. What are the key points raised in this article?
2. Do these key points raise any issues for you?
3. If so, how will you resolve these?

Your local NVQ Co-ordinator or your External Verifier may be of help to you.

Summary

Various assessment methods that can be used to generate evidence towards units D32 and D33 were discussed, with particular emphasis upon:

– the importance of generating evidence from workplace activities;
– accrediting prior learning and achievement;
– the need to plan assessments carefully in order to maximise their outcome;
– the need to record evidence in a meaningful and constructive way using a portfolio.

These issues are now summarised in the form of a checklist which can be used to review the evidence presented in the portfolio:

1. Is the evidence I am producing relevant to the performance criteria I am working towards?
2. Does my evidence cover all of the performance criteria?
3. Does my evidence meet the range?
4. Do I have the necessary underpinning knowledge?
5. Is this evidence up to date?

6. Can I demonstrate that the evidence has not been made up?
7. Is the evidence the product of my own work?
8. Have I maintained the confidentiality of my patient or client?
9. Have I laid out my evidence in a clear and consistent way?
10. Will my assessor be able to follow the evidence presented in my portfolio?

End of chapter activity: where are you now?

Using Figure 3.6, consider which of the stages of NVQ assessment you have reached. When you have looked at the diagram carefully, decide what action you are going to take.

- You may wish to turn to a page or section of this book in order to re-examine a particular issue concerning you.
- It may be that you are still undecided about whether to proceed with an NVQ Assessor Award, in which case another look at Chapters 2 and 4 may be helpful.

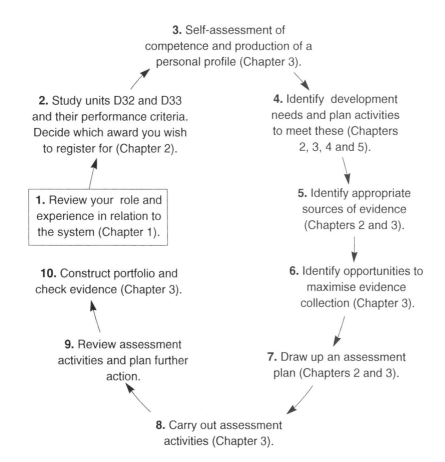

3. Self-assessment of competence and production of a personal profile (Chapter 3).

2. Study units D32 and D33 and their performance criteria. Decide which award you wish to register for (Chapter 2).

4. Identify development needs and plan activities to meet these (Chapters 2, 3, 4 and 5).

1. Review your role and experience in relation to the system (Chapter 1).

5. Identify appropriate sources of evidence (Chapters 2 and 3).

10. Construct portfolio and check evidence (Chapter 3).

6. Identify opportunities to maximise evidence collection (Chapter 3).

9. Review assessment activities and plan further action.

7. Draw up an assessment plan (Chapters 2 and 3).

8. Carry out assessment activities (Chapter 3).

Figure 3.6 **Where are you now? The stages of NVQ assessment**

- You may have registered with a centre but are unsure about what to do next. Chapter 3 will assist you here.
- Alternatively, you may have undertaken a self-assessment of competence and now require further help and guidance with the underpinning knowledge. Chapter 5 will help you with this.

Your NVQ Co-ordinator, your supervisor, or a friend undertaking an NVQ Assessor's Award may help clarify your thinking.

CHAPTER FOUR

Continuing assessor development

Introduction

Obtaining an assessor qualification isn't the end of the story. Many factors may influence the way in which an assessor works. Day (1994) highlighted these in a study which followed the work of a group of NVQ in Care assessors.

The study was carried out in two nursing homes over a period of 10 months. The researcher observed assessor interactions with NVQ candidates and surveyed assessor opinion in order to determine:

– how assessors perceived their role in the assessment of NVQs;
– what factors influenced assessor performance within the workplace;
– how assessors tackled the process of evaluation and the methods they used;
– how the working methods of assessors compared with the requirements of Awarding Bodies;
– the extent to which units D32 and D33 were a valid and reliable predictor of assessor performance.

This chapter reviews the findings of this study, and discusses the implications they may have for the continuing development of assessors.

Learning outcomes

At the end of this chapter the assessor student will be able to identify:

1. how practising assessors perceive their role in the assessment of NVQs;
2. the methods practising assessors use during workplace assessment;
3. the factors which may influence assessor performance within the workplace;

> ── Learning outcomes *continued* ─────────────
> **4.** the importance of continuing development and
> support for practising assessors.

Background to the study

All the assessors within the organisation studied were Registered
Nurses. With the exception of an education officer, who was a
Registered Nurse Tutor, none of the assessors had any experience in
training and development prior to their new role in the assessment
of NVQs in Care.

Before undertaking their new role, each assessor was required to
achieve TDLB unit D32. Each individual did this by developing a
portfolio which contained performance and supplementary evidence relating to the requirements of the relevant Awarding Body.

As a result of this activity each participant in the study had prior
knowledge of occupational standards for assessors, and had person-
ally experienced the process of NVQ assessment. Each participant
had also grown accustomed to an observer monitoring their performance whilst working with candidates.

Observation of assessor performance

A checklist of criteria relating to the occupational standards for first
line assessors was devised for the observation of assessments. This
was completed by the researcher during each assessment, and
completed by the assessor and candidate at the end of each assessment too.

The assessor and candidate were asked to record in confidence
whether the assessor's behaviour complied or did not comply with
the checklist criteria (see Figure 3.2). To reduce the possibility of bias,
it was decided that only areas of non-compliance or uncertainty
noted by the observer and at least two other recorders would be
reported.

In addition to the criteria checklist, the observer, assessor and
candidate were asked to indicate what factors, if any, might have
affected the outcome of any of the assessments observed. At the end
of each observation visit a report was submitted to the centre with
recommendations for action. Five observation visits were made in
all, covering a total of 14 assessments. The following findings were
reported:

1. Initial observation indicated that assessor performance did not

comply with the checklist criteria despite each assessor having previously demonstrated competence by the achievement of a first line Assessor Award (unit D32). It was felt this was due to a lack of opportunity to practise, brought about by delays in achieving full Accredited Centre status.

2. Subsequent observation visits indicated that after some initial guidance in the areas of action planning, questioning techniques and in providing feedback, assessor performance rapidly developed to the point where it met the majority of checklist criteria. This rapid improvement was noticed as early as the second observation round, indicating some support for the notion that lack of practice led to deterioration in assessor performance.

3. Confusion arose regarding the nature of leading questions. However, a tentative definition was put forward: *A leading question is probably one which (when posed by the assessor) either directly or indirectly gives the candidate the required answer, hence the candidate is led or directed.* – Day (1994). This definition appeared to register with the participants in the study, as demonstrated by the subsequent confidence shown in the use of a range of questioning skills and strategies.

4. Assessors throughout the study indicated a concern for the administrative requirements related to NVQ assessment. Assessors stated that these were time-consuming and repetitive. They were particularly concerned by the way NVQ procedures were constantly changing.

5. A trend emerged from the study. It was the degree to which evaluation had shifted from observation to written evidence. There appeared to be two reasons for this:

   (i) Assessors and candidates had worked together as friends and colleagues for many years. Therefore assessors had felt obliged to use written evidence in order to demonstrate to the External Verifier that they had overcome any personal bias when judging a colleague's competence.

   (ii) Assessors also felt that the setting of an essay or project would cause less disruption in the workplace than directly observing the candidate's performance.

Survey of assessor opinion

In addition to observation visits, the opinion of assessors regarding the necessary skills, knowledge and attributes required of the NVQ assessor was surveyed. A questionnaire asked assessors to identify factors that may affect their performance.

The results of this initial questionnaire were analysed. A series of 10 items relating to the knowledge, skills and attributes required of the assessor, together with 10 items pertaining to the factors affecting assessor performance, were identified.

These items were fed back to the assessors after each visit in a series of reiterative and successive questionnaires. Each one was asked to classify the items of each category in order of importance on a scale of 1 to 10, with 1 being the most important and 10 the least important. The findings are reported below.

The knowledge, skills and attributes of an NVQ assessor

1. Knowledge and skills

Participants in the study valued their professional skills above their evaluation skills. *Nursing and care delivery*, for example, was rated more highly than skills specific to assessment (see Table 4.1).

These findings were consistent with the requirements of the Joint Awarding Bodies who specify that assessors ought to be occupationally competent in the fields they evaluated. However, the Joint Awarding Bodies do not demand evidence of certification for occupational competence; this is an area of concern to professionals who are worried about the knowledge and skills base of some assessors in the residential care sector (see study activity 4, Chapter 1).

With regard to the knowledge characteristics that may be specific to the process of NVQ assessment, respondents indicated they highly valued the *principles of teaching* and the *principles of assessment* (see Table 4.1). This was confirmed by response to the skills category where *observing*, *listening* and *action planning* skills (subsets of the assessment process) were also rated highly (see Table 4.2).

Mid-range priority was allocated to knowledge of *how people learn* and the skills of *teaching* (see Tables 4.1 and 4.2). This supported the

Table 4.1
Knowledge characteristics: overall ranking

1.	Nursing and care delivery
2.	Candidate's potential
3.	Principles of teaching
4.	Principles of assessment
5.	How people learn
6.	NVQ terminology
7.	Anti-discriminatory practice
8.	NVQ policies and procedures
9.	Candidate's prior experience
10.	Supervisory management

idea that the process of *learning* was considered by assessors to be as important as that of *assessment*. In light of this finding, Awarding Bodies should, when determining quality assurance arrangements for centre approval, pay attention to the promotion of assessor standards relating to the processes of learning as well as to the process of assessment.

In addition to the findings outlined above, the reader's attention is drawn to the characteristics identified at the lower end of Tables 4.1 and 4.2. Of note was the limited value placed upon the knowledge of *supervisory management* and the skills of *supervision*. This was of note as the standards for Assessor Awards are drawn from Level 3 of the NCVQ framework which are defined as supervisory in nature.

Limited value was also placed upon *administration skills* and, although a large part of the NVQ assessor's role is taken up with administration, this could be explained by the way the participants perceived the assessment process as tedious and repetitive.

Finally, with regard to knowledge of a *candidate's prior experience* and knowledge of a *candidate's potential* (see Table 4.1), it was interesting to note that these characteristics scored so differently. However, subsequent analysis revealed that prior experience may be known *before* any appraisal had been initiated but was not necessarily an indication of success, whereas the potential to succeed could only be known *after* initiation of the evaluation and, given that all other items within this category were prerequisites of assessment, it was likely that these findings arose as a result of researcher error.

2. Attributes

The response of participants was interesting because characteristics traditionally associated with the role of the mentor (Darling, 1985; McMurray, 1986) were as highly valued as those which Awarding Bodies would ascribe to the role of the NVQ assessor.

Table 4.2 **Skills characteristics: overall ranking**	
1.	Nursing and care delivery
2.	Observing
3.	Listening
4.	Action planning
5.	Teaching
6.	Giving feedback
7.	Questioning
8.	Decision-making
9.	Supervising
10.	Administrating

For example, qualities such as *unbiased, approachable, committed, understanding* and *supportive* were placed above the middle of the scale, whereas characteristics associated with assessment and the assurance of quality, such as *accuracy* and *diligence,* were at the lower end of the scale (see Table 4.3).

At first glance it might be assumed that the above had implications on the quality of assessment within the organisation studied: there appeared to be a lack of recognition for the need to be accurate and diligent.

However, the characteristics respondents valued most were consistent with *process-based* approaches towards learning (see Table 4.3) which were also compatible with the requirements of delivering client-centred care (Burnard, 1984). It may be that respondents in this study were indicating a need for assessors to assume a caring and supportive role, one upon which candidates might model themselves. If this were the case, then a unique quality or condition for the assessor was recognised, a quality not appreciated by the requirements of the Training and Development Lead Body.

Factors influencing assessor performance

Assessors rated the following factors as those most likely to influence their performance:

– pressure of work;
– NVQ jargon;
– tiredness;
– the amount of paperwork.

Of these factors, pressure of work was rated the most important (see Table 4.4). This was consistent with anecdotal evidence which indicated that some organisations faced growing difficulty in implementing NVQ in Care awards due to the increasingly prohibitive cost of assessor replacement time. One way to overcome this might

*Table 4.3 **The attributes of the NVQ assessor***

1. Unbiased
2. Approachable
3. Committed
4. Understanding
5. Supportive
6. Praising
7. Helpful
8. Considerate
9. Accurate
10. Diligent

be to use supplementary methods of evidence collection, rather than direct observation of candidate performance. This was regarded as a more cost-effective use of time.

NVQ terminology

The effect of NVQ terminology – perceived as *NVQ jargon* – and its potential to alienate adult learners was described by Day (1993). If NVQ terminology influenced the assessment process and assessors were having difficulty interpreting standards, then there had to be doubts about the *reliability* of the assessment process.

To address this, the organisation under study established a regular pattern of meetings for assessors which proved useful in standardising approaches by ensuring a common understanding of the terminology involved. However, two further points arose:

1. more meetings meant an increase in assessor replacement time and corresponding increase in costs for NVQ assessment;
2. if interpretation of occupational standards was carried out at a local level, then there would appear to be no *national standard* for the assessment of NVQs in Care.

Work environment

Interestingly, assessors did not rate *work environment* as a significant factor in influencing their performance, this despite frequent interruptions during assessment of candidates. The observer noted, for example, telephone calls or requests for assistance. It may be that the observer recorded these in anticipation of a detrimental effect, but in reality they had little, as both assessor and candidate were already accustomed to these as part of their normal workplace culture.

Not one of the respondents indicated that the research process influenced the assessments they undertook. This was also a feature of the reports completed by assessors and candidates. The explana-

Table 4.4
Factors
affecting
assessor
performance

1. Pressure of work
2. NVQ jargon
3. Tiredness
4. The amount of paperwork
5. Home and personal commitments
6. Work environment
7. Too many candidates
8. Inadequate training and development
9. Unresponsive candidate
10. Lack of support from colleagues

tion could be that participants had experienced observation by a third party for their Assessor Award.

Direct or indirect researcher influence upon the observed performance may be regarded as a potential danger for any observational research and, although it is not claimed to have been totally eliminated from this study, it seems likely in view of participants' responses that it had been minimised.

Methods used by NVQ assessors

A significant shift away from the use of direct observation of candidate performance to the use of supplementary methods of appraisal appeared to have taken place. The most obvious example of this approach related to the assessment of the 'O' Unit. Such methods included oral exchanges, the use of evidence generated from study days and workshops, and the setting of specific projects and assignments.

The main reasons for this shift appeared to be:

- the effective use of an assessor's time (it was easier to set an essay or a project than to observe a candidate at work);
- a need to legitimise the evaluation process (candidates known to the assessor for some time were set additional written work in an attempt to demonstrate greater objectivity to the External Verifier);
- responding to the needs of candidates (some candidates preferred written assessments to direct observation).

This shift in approach had implications for the quality assurance of the assessment process. For example:

- evidence produced at a workshop may be the product of several candidates' work and it may not be a true record of individual performance;
- written work relating to the requirements of the 'O' Unit may not give a true indication of a candidate's behaviour towards a client.

Such issues might only be resolved by ensuring that evidence from a variety of different sources is used to validate the assessment outcome. However, such an approach may be more time-consuming than direct observation.

Assessor perceptions and demands of Awarding Bodies

With a shift away from direct observation of performance to the use of supplementary methods of evidence collection, the assessors in the study were no longer undertaking first line assessor roles.

The first line assessor was defined by the Training and Development Lead Body as an individual who would normally directly supervise and assess the candidate within the workplace – for example, in the case of this study, a Staff Nurse who normally directly observed the performance of the NVQ candidate while undertaking care activities.

However, the experience of assessors in the study led them to develop a system of evaluation closer to the second line assessor role. This appeared in complete contrast to the guidelines laid down by the Joint Awarding Bodies, prescribing that at least 80% of any assessment should be conducted by direct observation of candidate performance within the workplace.

This change in practice would have cost implications for these assessors, as the Awarding Body demanded certificated competence of assessors in their new role, occasioning additional costs by further assessment for the D33 or second line Assessor Award.

Occupational standards and assessor performance

Although each participant had achieved a recognised Assessor Award before the study, initial observation indicated assessors did not comply with Training and Development Lead Body criteria for first line assessors. This was largely thought to be due to lack of practice because of delays in gaining full Accredited Centre status.

After an initial period of guidance, assessor performance rapidly developed beyond the point specified by the Training and Development Lead Body, to a point where concern for the process of learning and new assessor roles was developed.

On achievement of full Accredited Centre status, assessor performance rapidly grew beyond the specifications of the Training and Development Lead Body, after an initial period of guidance followed by setting up an assessor peer support group. Figure 4.1 shows the stages of development of the assessor's expertise. Progression was dependent upon hands-on experience, individual guidance by the education officer and the support of other assessors.

Such a model questioned the validity of occupational standards for assessors as a reliable predictor of long-term assessor performance. The prescriptive nature of these standards disregarded a person's unique experience and ability to go beyond the minimal requirements laid down by the Training and Development Lead Body.

The standards also ignored the potential for the assessor's performance to 'tail off'. In the case of this study, this was caused by lack of opportunity to practise, but could also have been brought about by

Expert assessor:
Development of assessment role beyond that identified by the TDLB*.
Demonstrates advanced questioning skills.
Has concern for the learning process.

Development phase:
Practice refined; developed by assessment experience and
enhanced by peer review and support.

Non-compliance:
Reduced opportunity for practice.

Competent assessor:
As defined by TDLB* standards.

Beginner:
Induction and assessment to
TDLB* standards.

* Training and
Development
Lead Body

*Figure 4.1 **The stages of NVQ assessor development***

other factors such as pressure of work, tiredness or the quantity and tedium of assessment administration.

Given these findings, it is recommended that awarding bodies place greater emphasis upon the need for continuing assessor development in their centre approval guidelines. It is also recommended that awarding bodies be more responsive to organisations who wish to become approved NVQ centres, as delays in the approval process affect the outcomes of any staff development activity undertaken.

Assessors' continuing development needs: case study

To meet continuing development needs of assessors, staff within the organisation studied developed the following systems.

1. Formation of an Assessment Board

An Assessment Board was established within the centre. Its membership included the organisation's principal budget holder, the NVQ Co-ordinator, an assessor and an NVQ candidate. The Assessment Board co-ordinated the appointment and development of assessors within the centre and determined programmes and resources for their future development (see Table 4.5).

Table 4.5 **Terms of reference: Assessment Board**

Prepare and develop systems and policies relating to the process of assessment in order to gain, and then sustain, approval as an Accredited NVQ Assessment Centre.

Appoint workplace assessors and Internal Verifiers as necessary, and advise Awarding Bodies of their registration and ongoing development.

Ensure equality of access for anyone wishing to undertake NVQ assessment.

Provide a system by which NVQ candidates may appeal against the outcomes of NVQ assessment.

Receive reports from assessors on standards relating to the inputs, process and outcomes of NVQ assessment and relating to their overall effectiveness. Take appropriate action.

Submit an annual report to the Awarding Bodies describing local developments relating to the assessment of NVQs.

To act upon the recommendations of Awarding Bodies to accommodate any future changes in the process of NVQ assessment.

2. Formation of an Assessors' Panel

Chaired by the NVQ Co-ordinator, this committee reported to the Assessment Board on activities relating to the process of assessment. It identified the development needs of assessors within the centre (see Table 4.6) who were expected to attend this panel at least twice a year. If an assessor did not comply with this criterion, he or she was struck off the 'live register' until a personal action plan for development could be implemented by the NVQ Co-ordinator.

3. Performance reviews for assessors

Assessors underwent a periodic review of performance conducted by a member of the Assessment Board in order to determine a personal action plan for their development (see Figure 4.2). A 'live register' of assessors was kept, which required periodic updating and amending by the Centre.

Table 4.6 **Terms of reference: assessors' panel**

Discuss reports concerning the monitoring of NVQ assessment and the effectiveness of the NVQ assessment process.

Identify deficiencies and discrepancies in the process of NVQ assessment. Notify the Assessment Board accordingly.

Identify changes and developments in the practice of NVQ assessment and make appropriate recommendations for assessor development to the Assessment Board.

Individual performance review for NVQ assessors

1. Personal details:

Assessor's name: Qualifications:

Locality: Telephone Number:

2. Review Criteria: **Yes**   **No**

i. Is the assessor familiar with policies for NVQ assessment? ☐ ☐

ii. Is the assessor able to demonstrate an ability to promote anti-discriminatory practice? ☐ ☐

iii. Does the assessor regularly attend Assessor Panel meetings? ☐ ☐

iv. Does the assessor participate in the monitoring and review of NVQ assessors' performance? ☐ ☐

v. Can the assessor clearly identify their own development needs in relation to their role as an assessor? ☐ ☐

3. Outcomes of the review process (delete as appropriate):

(a) Accept continuance as a practising assessor
(b) Further development is required

4. Agreed action plan:

Signed (assessor):   Date:

Signed (Assessment Board member):   Date:

N.B. Copy to assessor, submit to Assessment Board for approval, then retain in a secure file.

Figure 4.2 **Individual performance review for assessors**

4. Assessor development workshops

Assessor development workshops were instigated to examine the role of the second line assessor and coaching and guidance skills. The content of the workshops depended upon action plans arising from the periodic review of assessor performance. An example of the 'questioning skills' and 'giving feedback' workshops arising from the study is presented in Table 4.7.

Table 4.7 **Workshops for the development of assessor questioning and feedback skills**

Session 1: Asking questions At the end of the session the assessor will be able to:	Session 2: Responding, challenging and giving feedback At the end of the session the assessor will be able to:
1. outline the usefulness of different questioning techniques in establishing and maintaining an interaction;	1. state ways in which listening and responding can affect interpersonal communication;
2. identify the main types of questions used during a conversation, e.g. 'closed', 'open', 'leading', 'probing' etc.;	2. state ways in which feedback can be given in a constructive manner;
3. describe other methods available in clarifying the meaning of a conversation, e.g. 'paraphrasing', 'reflecting' etc.;	3. describe the styles of responding as outlined by Carl Rogers, e.g. 'evaluative', 'interpretative', 'supportive', 'probing' and 'understanding';
4. demonstrate an ability to use different clarification and questioning techniques in order to establish and maintain an interaction and to elicit data.	4. define *assertiveness* and identify ways in which a person's feelings and opinions may be expressed;
	5. make understanding responses rather than evaluative ones during an interaction;
	6. make use of specific techniques to enable expression of own feelings and opinions during an interaction, e.g. use of 'cracked record', 'compromising', 'time out', 'content-process shift'.

5. D32 and D33 as preparation for becoming an assessor

In addition to satisfying requirements for continuing assessor development, it was recommended that individuals who were undergoing initial preparation to become assessors undertake a programme combining both the first line and second line assessor role. Future assessors would obtain a certificate of competence in both units D32 and D33 of the Training and Development Lead Body awards.

Summary

This chapter has considered the following findings of a study relating to the role and performance of the NVQ assessor.

1. Assessors were concerned with the process of learning, which they valued as much as the process of assessment.
2. Assessors were concerned about the tedious and repetitive

75

administrative requirements for assessment, to the extent where it was felt this could influence their performance.

3. A lack of opportunity to practise caused by delays in centre approval, together with pressure of work, NVQ jargon and general tiredness may influence the performance of NVQ assessors.

4. The roles of first line and second line assessors (as defined by the Training and Development Lead Body) were perhaps not a true reflection of assessment practice within a care environment. First line assessors in the study appeared to favour supplementary methods of evidence-collection in an attempt to ensure cost-effective use of their time.

5. Assessors also favoured supplementary methods in order to 'legitimise' the appraisal of candidates known to them as colleagues for some time.

6. Standards defined by the Training and Development Lead Body did not always provide a valid and reliable predictor of assessor performance within a care environment because they did not take into account the potential 'tailing off' of assessor performance due to lack of opportunity to practise.

In view of these findings it was recommended that accredited NVQ centres give careful consideration to:

– the provision of assessor training that equally highlighted the *process of learning* as well as the *process of assessment*: these programmes should also recognise the diverse evaluation activities of those working within the care environment;
– the continuing development of practising assessors: by paying attention to the quality assurance and support systems required for the continuing education and update of assessors.

The end of chapter activity deals with these two issues.

 End of chapter activity: preparation and development

With the help of the guidelines in the chapter on study skills, search out and appraise the following articles:

Day, M. (1993). NVQ Assessment for Care Assistants. *Nursing Standard.* Vol. 7, No. 29, pp35–38.

Day, M. (1994). The needs of individuals undertaking an NVQ in Care. *NVQ/SVQ Focus and Care Standard.* Vol. 2, No. 4, pp30,31.

Day, M. (1995). An Evaluation of the Role and Performance of the NVQ Assessor within an Independent Health Care Organisation. Part One: A Summary Account. *NVQ/SVQ Focus and*

Care Standard. Vol. 2, No. 7, pp31,32.

Day, M. (1995). An Evaluation of the Role and Performance of the NVQ Assessor within an Independent Health Care Organisation. Part Two: Observing the Role and Performance of the NVQ Assessor. *NVQ/SVQ Focus and Care Standard.* Vol. 2, No. 8, pp36–39.

Day, M. (1995). An Evaluation of the Role and Performance of the NVQ Assessor within an Independent Health Care Organisation. Part Three: Assessor Perceptions of their Role and the Factors which may influence this. *NVQ/SVQ Focus and Care Standard.* Vol. 2, No. 9, pp40–42.

Now answer the following questions:

1. What are the key points raised in these articles?
2. Do these key points raise any issues for you as an assessor student?
3. If so, how will you resolve these?

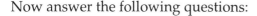

Your NVQ Co-ordinator and External Verifier may be of help to you in answering these questions. You may wish to record your answers in the Learning Record (see Appendix 2).

CHAPTER FIVE

Study skills

Introduction

This book induces an active process: it aims to encourage the seeking of new information and applying this new knowledge to working practice. This chapter covers the process of *seeking out*, *learning* and *applying information*.

```
┌─── Learning outcomes ──────────────────────────┐
│ After studying this chapter the assessor student will be
│ able to:
│ 1. conduct a library search in order to identify
│    appropriate NVQ literature;
│ 2. systematically read and review appropriate NVQ
│    literature;
│ 3. construct a card index system to record appropriate
│    NVQ literature.
└────────────────────────────────────────────────┘
```

Adult learning

Young people grasp, develop and try out new ideas very fast – often at an alarming rate! Unfortunately, as people mature their capacity to absorb the same amount of information often diminishes. The adult learner can overcome this by drawing upon a greater knowledge and life experience. New learning becomes easier if it is made interesting and relevant, particularly if it is appropriately connected to the world of work.

The adult learner needs to try out ideas, test them out and apply them to everyday experience before retaining them. How people do this varies: some take immediate action and then reflect upon their experience; others might think carefully and plan a strategy before acting. Whatever the starting point, research into adult learning has shown that mature students often move through a common cycle of learning (see Figure 5.1).

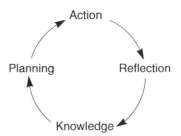

Figure 5.1
Adult learning cycle

In practice it would be more realistic to picture this process as a *spiral* rather than a *circle* as learning never ceases. Each new skill or piece of knowledge acquired enables us to plan ahead, contributes something to draw upon when we encounter new problems or situations. Much of the time we are not conscious of this process.

The portfolio

This is the process that takes place when compiling a portfolio of evidence, though in a more self-aware and reflective way. For example, the portfolio and its contents show thinking about:

1. what the assessor student is trying to do;
2. the most effective way to do this;
3. what is needed to be known in order to do this;
4. how well the assessor student is succeeding;
5. why one particular approach to assessment works but another does not;
6. what would be done differently in future;
7. how the assessor student demonstrates to the assessor that the criteria and range required have been met.

Using a library

The library is an essential resource for anyone undertaking an NVQ Assessor Award. Using the library helps to gather relevant information and also provides a quiet and peaceful environment in which to study – quite a luxury for those who lead busy lives!

Some may be lucky and have easy access to the local school of nursing library or have access to the public library service. If not already a member of a library it is worth joining one which will serve specified needs: not all libraries provide specialist advice on health care and some charge for accessing this type of information. Most libraries offer the following:

1. books on long- and short-term loan;
2. periodicals and journals, e.g. *NVQ/SVQ Focus* and *Care Standard* or *Nursing Standard*;

3. bibliographies: a list of past and current publications;
4. inter-library loans;
5. government publications;
6. dictionaries;
7. audio-visual equipment, e.g. video or audio tapes;
8. computer search facilities using CD ROM;
9. photographic and photocopying services.

All library information is catalogued systematically whether it be books, journals, newspapers etc. Accessing this information might appear complex, but libraries have established systems for this.

Manual storage systems

The Dewey System is most commonly used for books in libraries. This system allocates three-figure numbers to each category of books within a library. For example, *000* for generalities, *100* for Philosophy and related disciplines, *200* for Religion and so on. Many of these categories have so many items that the category number is broken down into parts or sub-sets. This facilitates storage and retrieval.

For example, *800* corresponds to Literature, but American Literature in English is categorised under *810*, while English and Anglo-Saxon Literature is classified under *820*, etc. (This type of arrangement will be familiar: NVQ units are broken down into elements, and then into performance criteria.)

A *library card index* is used in conjunction with the Dewey system. The information is listed either under the subject title, or the author's surname. The card corresponding to the book wanted will carry a Dewey number. This number serves to locate the book on the shelves. Alternatively, a microfiche machine can be used to find the volume required. Again, information is recorded under subject or author's name with corresponding Dewey number.

Study activity 14

Visit your local library and familiarise yourself with the Dewey numbers associated with your subject area. Remember you are looking at general categories such as *Education and Training* or *Post-16 Education* or *Human Resource Development*. It is within these general categories that you are likely to find the specific subjects of *Competence-based training* or *National Vocational Qualifications*. The librarian will be able to assist you with this activity.

Computerised storage systems

Computers can help locate a journal article or book relating to the subject studied. You can use:

- CD ROM for research and journal articles; or
- OPAC (On-line Public Access Catalogue) for books.

CD ROM

CD ROM searches the entries on a compact disc via a personal computer. This is a very powerful and quick way of identifying information required. One of the most useful discs in the context of care is CINAHL – the *Cumulated Index of Nursing and Allied Health Literature.*

Most libraries with CD ROM facilities provide training, and step-by-step advice on how to use the disc and the computer. To use CD ROM, a disc is inserted into the computer disc drive, the appropriate command is keyed to load the disc onto the computer, then it is a matter of following the commands on the screen.

Clear and succinct search terms (key words) have to be entered into the computer. The starting point is to identify the words which might appear in the title of an article. For example, in searching for information about 'The NVQ in care value base', the words *NVQ* and *value base* are the most productive, whereas *the* or *in* will throw up several thousand sources of information, as they are used in the title of virtually all journal articles.

It is therefore necessary to refine and limit the key words employed in a search. It is suggested this is done before using CINAHL, so as not to get side-tracked! Once the information required has been tracked down, the computer can be instructed to print it out on paper (the *hard copy*). This hard copy is a useful reference to help retrieve any of the articles identified.

OPAC

OPAC will help to locate books in the library. It has an author and subject index, plus a facility to enter key words to focus an information search more accurately.

Other sources of information

Dictionaries, encyclopedias, directories, handbooks and manuals are all useful resources when seeking out concise information or for clarification of meaning. NVQ candidates will want to read articles relating to care activities in journals, magazines or newspapers. At times it may be desirable to review several articles on a particular topic, either from different sources or across a period of time. If the articles are not available at the local library, then they may be obtained through inter-library loan (some libraries charge for this service).

Study activity 15

Visit your local library and familiarise yourself with the relevant journals for your topic area. Seek out the following article:

Nursing Times (1989). View from the Front Line. *Nursing Times.* Vol. 85, No. 7, pp32–33.

Now answer the following:

1. What is the main focus of the article?
2. How many respondents were there?
3. What was the belief which united the auxiliaries?
4. Is the title 'support worker' one they liked? Give an example to back your answer.
5. How many commentators suggested they would join the RCN?
6. In your own words, sum up the views expressed.

Reading

Visiting a library often is an enjoyable experience. Reading, however, requires organisation. A student is not expected to read everything written about a single topic, therefore it is very important to decide which book or article is the most important to read.

Different people adopt different strategies for reading. It is important to identify needs. It is useful to begin by asking:

1. Why am I reading this book or article?
2. In what way is it relevant?
3. What am I getting from it that is new to me?

Getting started

There is a simple method for getting the best out of reading. Known as the SQ3R method (Williams, 1989), it stands for *Survey, Question, Read, Recall, Review.*

Survey

In the case of a book, scanning the contents page and index will reveal what can be expected; for an article, scanning the abstract, introduction and summary. Noting headings, sub-headings, bold print and italics, then reading the first sentence of each paragraph will provide an overview of the content.

Question

Identifying what questions the article will be able to answer once it has been read in detail. The survey will assist in formulating the questions.

Read

Having completed the above, it is time to read carefully and find the answers to any questions. This done, there is little point in reading the rest of the book or article in detail. End of chapter summaries may help.

Recall

By trying to answer all questions without looking at the book or referring to notes will show what has been learned and what has to be concentrated upon.

Review

Reading the relevant sections in the book or article again checks out the accuracy of the information gained.

Effective reading

Effective reading is not about reading at speed, but is about being flexible and purposeful. There are techniques to enhance reading skills and learning, including the following:

1. identifying the purpose for the reading without getting side-tracked!
2. seeking out the relevant, and therefore the most important information;
3. evaluating the content for its relevance to prior knowledge;
4. breaking off at intervals to reflect on understanding the content;
5. making a conscious effort to interpret the text and draw conclusions;
6. making brief notes to aid memory.

Adding comments and evaluations to the notes taken, getting into the habit of writing summaries and comparing these with the summaries of colleagues, making sure the source of information is recorded, noting the author, date of publication, journal or book title etc. are all part of effective reading skills. Details of books are recorded as follows:

> Day, M., Basford, L. and Cooper, M. (1996). *The Role of the Health Care Worker: NVQs and the 'O' Unit*. Campion Press. Edinburgh.

Journal articles should be recorded in the style:

> Day, M. (1993). NVQ Assessment for care assistants. *Nursing Standard*. Vol. 7, No. 29, pp35–38.

Maintaining a card index system

Recording the information gained from reading onto index cards is a good idea. These can be stored in a box with alphabetical dividers. The information recorded should include:

1. details of the book or article;
2. how it fits into the area of study;
3. any useful quotes: these should be in italics or between 'quote' marks, with a note of the page number;
4. a brief summary of the article: the CD ROM printout could be useful here!
5. your own evaluation of the article;
6. any further sources of information the article may refer to.

There is no definite style for this, but a consistent approach is important.

Organising a card index system

It is useful to organise information into study categories. For example, the following headings could be practical to an assessor for NVQs in Care.

1. The organisation and structure of health and social care in the UK.
2. The role of the health care worker.
3. Understanding NVQs.
4. NVQ assessment.
5. The 'O' Unit or value base.

It is also worth allocating a separate card to every item of information: these can then be grouped in a variety of ways. When the information gathered is of value in relation to several categories it will then be easier to cross-reference what has been read.

For example, it may be desirable to reference *NCVQ guidelines and criteria* under sections 3 and 4 of the index (see above). This could seem laborious, but it is worth while in the long run, particularly when the time comes to identify evidence towards the Assessor Award!

Summary

This chapter has focused on adult learning, study skills, the use of library facilities and the different methods of searching for information. Methods for effective reading and recording of information have also been discussed, and a mechanism for indexing appropriate literature has been suggested.

This chapter explained how to use the library and organise reading material in a meaningful way so as to enable completion of under-pinning knowledge requirements for the NVQ Assessor Award.

Learning never stops, it is a constant feature of adult life. A helpful list of recommended reading is provided on the next few pages. Bon voyage!

Recommended reading

Health and social care within the UK

Arber, S. and Ginn, J. (1990). The meaning of informed care: gender and the contribution of elderly people. *Ageing and Society*. Vol. 10, No. 4, pp429–454.

Barry, N. (1990). *Welfare.* Milton Keynes: Open University.

Basford, L. and Slevin, O. (1995). *Theory and Practice of Nursing.* Edinburgh: Campion Press.

Benner, P. (1989). *The Primacy of Caring: Stress and coping in health and illness.* Addison Wesley.

Cox, C. (1983). *Sociology: An introduction for nurses, midwives and health visitors.* Kent: Butterworths.

Department of Health (1989). *Caring for People – Community Care in the next decade and beyond.* CM 849. London: HMSO.

Department of Health (1989). *Working for Patients.* CM 555. London: HMSO.

Department of Health (1991). *The Health of the Nation.* London: HMSO.

DHSS (1983). *Elderly People in the Community.* London: HMSO.

DHSS (1988). *Community Care: Agenda for action – Report to the Secretary of State for Social Services.* Sir Roy Griffiths. London: HMSO.

DHSS (1990). *People first – Community Care in Northern Ireland.* London: HMSO.

HMSO (1990). *National Health Service and Community Care Act.* London: HMSO.

The role of the health care worker

Brooks, J. and Rutter, J. (1990). More than a support. *Nursing Times.* Vol. 86, No. 5, pp64–65.

Care Sector Consortium (1992). *National Occupational Standards for Care.* London: HMSO.

Chapman, P. (1990). We can do that. *Nursing Times.* Vol. 6, No. 16, p34.

Chudley, P. (1988). More of the same. *Nursing Times.* Vol. 84, No. 29, p19.

Davies, T. (1989). More questions than answers. *Nursing Times.* Vol. 85, No. 7, pp28–29.

Day, M., Basford, L. and Cooper M. (1996). *The Role of the Health Care Worker: NVQs and the 'O' Unit.* Edinburgh: Campion Press.

Fardell, J. (1989). Short cut or short change? *Nursing Times.* Vol. 85, No. 7, pp30–31.

Gaze, H. (1990). A glimpse into the future. *Nursing Times.* Vol. 86, No. 16, pp28–31.

Hardie, M. (1987). A special kind of person. *Nursing Times.* Vol. 83, No. 10, pp26–27.

Hughes, P. (1992). The implications of NVQs for nursing. *Nursing Standard.* Vol. 7, No. 19, p29.

Johnston, C. (1989). Who is the support worker? *Nursing Times.* Vol. 85, No. 7, p26.

Mackie Bailey, S. (1991). Preparing health care assistants. *Nursing Standard.* Vol. 5, No. 24, pp38–40.

Malby, R. (1990). Vocational support. *Nursing Times.* Vol. 86, No. 16, pp31–32.

Nursing Times (1989). View from the frontline. *Nursing Times.* Vol. 85, No. 7, pp32–33.

Robinson, J. (1990). The role of the support worker in the health care team. *Nursing Times.* Vol. 86, No. 37, pp61–63.

Storey, L. (1991). Points of view. *Nursing Standard.* Vol. 5, No. 24, p43.

Understanding NVQs

Care Sector Consortium National Occupational Standards for Care. July 1992.

Care Standard (1993). Approval of assessment arrangements to offer NVQs in Care. *Care Standard.* Vol. 1, No. 6, pp8–9.

McCrory, R. (1992). Understanding National Vocational Qualifications and Standards: A handbook. Lancs: Parthenon.

National Council Vocational Qualifications (1992). *Brief Guide NVQs and Work.* London: NCVQ.

National Council Vocational Qualifications (1992). *NVQ Notes Access and Equal Opportunities.* London: NCVQ.

National Council Vocational Qualifications (1992). *Brief Guide NVQ.* London: NCVQ.

National Council Vocational Qualifications (1992). *Brief Guide NVQs and Careers Guidance.* London: NCVQ.

National Health Service Training Directorate (1993). *25 Questions and Answers on National Vocational Qualifications.* Bristol: NHSTD.

Stoten, T. (1992). *A Manager's Guide to the NVQs in Care.* Suffolk Training and Enterprise Council and the Registered Nursing Homes Association.

Stoten, T. (1992). *A Carer's Guide to the NVQs in Care.* Suffolk Training and Enterprise Council and the Registered Nursing Homes Association.

Waxman, L. (1993). A look at centre approval, quality and the D Units. *Care Standard.* Vol. 1, No. 10, p8.

Whitear, G. (1993). *The NVQ Handbook: A Guide to Career Success.* London: Pitman.

NVQ assessment

Central Council for the Education and Training of Social Workers (1990). *Assessment in Social Care: Trainer's manual.* North West Regional Training Unit.

Day, M. (1992). Quality training for health care assistants. *Nursing Standard.* Vol. 6, No. 24, pp32–34.

Day, M. (1993). NVQ assessment for care assistants. *Nursing Standard.* Vol. 7, No. 29, pp35–38.

Day, M. (1994). The needs of individuals undertaking an NVQ in Care. *NVQ/SVQ Focus and Care Standard.* Vol. 2, No. 4, pp30,31.

Day, M. (1995). An evaluation of the role and performance of the NVQ assessor within an independent health care organisation. Part One: a summary account. *NVQ/SVQ Focus and Care Standard.* Vol. 2, No. 7, pp31,32.

Day, M. (1995). An evaluation of the role and performance of the NVQ assessor within an independent health care organisation. Part Two: observing the role and performance of the NVQ assessor. *NVQ/SVQ Focus and Care Standard.* Vol. 2, No. 8, pp36–39.

Day, M. (1995). An evaluation of the role and performance of the NVQ assessor within an independent health care organisation. Part Three: assessor perceptions of their role and the factors which may influence this. *NVQ/SVQ Focus and Care Standard.* Vol. 2, No. 9, pp40–42.

Joint Awarding Bodies (1992). *National Vocational Qualifications in Care: Notes on assessment and verification.* London: J.A.B.

Mathias, P. (1993). Assessment requirements, knowledge and the log sheet. *Care Standard.* Vol. 1, No. 6, pp6,7.

National Council for Vocational Qualifications (1992). *NVQs and Prior Learning Action Pack.* London: NCVQ.

National Council for Vocational Qualifications (1995). *NVQ Criteria and Guidance.* London: NCVQ.

National Health Service Training Directorate (1991). *Occupational Standards for NVQ Assessors Training Resource Pack.* Bristol: NHSTD.

Royal Society of Arts (1991). *Accreditation of Prior Achievement.* Coventry: Royal Society of Arts Examination Board.

Stoten, T. (1992). *NVQs in Care: A guide for assessors.* Suffolk Training and Enterprise Council and the Registered Nursing Homes Association.

Training and Development Lead Body (1992). *National Standards for Training and Development.* Sheffield, Moorfoot: Employment Department.

The 'O' unit or value base

Burnard, P. (1985). *Learning Human Skills.* London: Heinemann.

Centre for Policy on Ageing (1990). *Community Life: A code of practice for Community Care.*

Hewitt, F.S. (1981). Introduction to communication. *Nursing Times.* Vol. 77, No. 4, pp9–12.

Hewitt, F.S. (1981). Non-verbal communication. *Nursing Times.* Vol. 77, No. 13, pp9–12.

Hewitt, F.S. (1981). Role and the presentation of the self. *Nursing Times.* Vol. 77, No. 22, pp17–20.

HMSO (1966). *Local Government Act.* London: HMSO.

HMSO (1976). *Race Relations Act.* London: HMSO.

HMSO (1983). *Mental Health Act.* London: HMSO.

HMSO (1986). *Data Protection Act.* London: HMSO.

HMSO (1987). *Access to Personal Files Act.* London: HMSO.

HMSO (1990). *Medical Records Act.* London: HMSO.

HMSO (1990). *National Health Service and Community Care Act.* London: HMSO.

HMSO (1991). *Citizen's Charter*. London: HMSO.

Local Government Management Board (1992). *Quality of Care*. Ref. SS0045X1. LGMB.

Local Health Authority. *The Patient's Charter*.

MacMillan, S. The bridge-builders' guide. *Nursing Times*. Vol. 77, No. 4, pp151–152.

MacMillan, S. The bridge-builders' guide. What's in a word? *Nursing Times*. Vol. 77, No. 9, pp354–355.

MacMillan, S. The bridge-builders' guide. Getting through without words. *Nursing Times*. Vol. 77, No. 13, pp554–555.

MacMillan, S. The bridge-builders' guide. Spacing and touching and hugging. *Nursing Times*. Vol. 77, No. 18, pp788–789.

Miller, M. (1984). Stop, look and listen. *Nursing Mirror*. Vol. 158, No. 3, pp40–41.

Nelson-Jones, R. (1991). *Human Relationship Skills*. London: Cassell.

UK Central Council for Nursing and Midwifery (1992). *Code of Professional Conduct*. London: UKCC.

The Learning Record

What is a Learning Record?

A completed Learning Record can provide evidence that there is enough *underpinning knowledge* for a particular NVQ Unit. In this book it is related to the study activities for the NVQ Assessor's Award offered in each chapter.

When completed, the Learning Record is submitted to the assessor who will ask questions relating to it. For example, whether it was all the assessor student's own work, how it relates to the elements and performance criteria concerned, as well as questions about the content of the material presented.

How do I keep a Learning Record?

To keep a Learning Record, carry out the following steps:

1. *Identify a strategy to answer the study activity considered:*
   relevant information has to be sought out, read, appraised and recorded in a meaningful way. (Chapter 5 discussed these skills and provided a reading list.) In addition it may be good to discuss the study activity with a more experienced colleague or to attend a study day for updating purposes.
2. *Identify what you have learned by giving an answer to the study activity:*
   taking into account any reading and discussions.
3. *Apply what you have learned to your practice:*
   by indicating how new knowledge will be used to assess candidates.
4. *Identify the evidence you will put forward to demonstrate you have the appropriate underpinning knowledge:*
   this will need to be discussed with the assessor, but it may include a record of any reading (see Chapter 5), notes taken, copies of diagrams produced by the assessor student and any certificates of learning received.

What does a Learning Record look like?

An example of a Learning Record and how it might be completed follows. A blank Learning Record is also provided on page 96. The blank Learning Record could serve to note down answers to the study activities in this book. It is a good idea to photocopy it (making extra copies in case of mistakes). Good luck!

Learning Record

Candidate's name: Awarding Body no.:

Centre name: Assessor:

Page number: This will help you and your assessor to identify
                 which study activity you are referring to in this book.

1. Your strategy for learning:

You could seek relevant information from the library (see Chapter 5) or consult a colleague.

Or you could attend a study day relating to the area being tested.

2. Your response to the study activity:

Answer the questions listed in each study activity, based on the information you have gathered.

3. How you will apply your knowledge to assessing your candidates:

State how your new knowledge will be applied to the assessment of your candidates.

4. Evidence you can put forward:

List sources of evidence that show you have the appropriate underpinning knowledge. For example, a record of your reading, a copy of any notes you have made, or any study day attendance certificates.

This evidence has to be cross-referenced to the appropriate element and performance criteria of the 'D' Units – as you did in the accreditation of prior learning exercise in Chapter 3.

5. Assessor's comments:

Your assessor will need to record whether it is agreed you have the necessary underpinning knowledge, and confirm which element and performance criteria this relates to. Your assessor could do this by recording the questions asked and your response to them (possibly using the space provided and continuing on the back of your Learning Record).

Signed (candidate):   Date:

Signed (assessor):   Date:

NB
please
photo-
copy for
your
own use

Learning Record

Candidate's name: Awarding Body no.:

Centre name: Assessor:

Page number:

1. Your strategy for learning:

2. Your response to the study activity:

3. How you will apply your knowledge to assessing your candidates:

4. Evidence you can put forward:

5. Assessor's comments:

Signed (candidate):   Date:

Signed (assessor):   Date:

References

Burnard, P. (1984). Paradigms for progress. *Senior Nurse*. Vol. 1, No. 38, pp24–25.

Care Sector Consortium (1992). *National Occupational Standards for Care*. London: HMSO.

Central Council for the Education and Training of Social Workers (1990). *Assessment in Social Care: Trainer's manual*. North West Regional Training Unit.

Chapman, P. (1990). We can do that. *Nursing Times*. Vol. 6, No. 16, p34.

Chudley, P. (1988). More of the same. *Nursing Times*. Vol. 84, No. 29, p19.

Confederation British Industry (1989). *Towards a Skills Revolution: Report of the Vocational Education and Training Task Force*. London: CBI.

Darling, L.W. (1985). Mentors and mentoring. *Nurse Education*. Vol. 10, No. 6, pp18,19.

Davies, J. (1993). The comparative cost of assessor training. *NVQ/SVQ Focus*. Vol. 1, No. 3, pp24,25.

Davies, T. (1989). More questions than answers. *Nursing Times*. Vol. 85, No. 7, pp28,29.

Day, M. (1992). Quality training for health care assistants. *Nursing Standard*. Vol. 6, No. 24, pp32–34.

Day, M. (1993). NVQ assessment for care assistants. *Nursing Standard*. Vol. 7, No. 29, pp35–38.

Day, M. (1994). *An Evaluation of the Role and Performance of the NVQ Assessor within an Independent Health Care Organisation* [M.Ed. Dissertation]. Bangor: University College North Wales.

Day, M. (1995). An evaluation of the role and performance of the NVQ assessor within an independent health care organisation. Part

One: a summary account. *NVQ/SVQ Focus and Care Standard*. Vol. 2, No. 7, pp31,32.

Day, M. (1995). An evaluation of the role and performance of the NVQ assessor within an independent health care organisation. Part Two: observing the role and performance of the NVQ assessor. *NVQ/ SVQ Focus and Care Standard*. Vol. 2, No. 8, pp36–39.

Day, M. (1995). An evaluation of the role and performance of the NVQ assessor within an independent health care organisation. Part Three: assessor perceptions of their role and the factors which may influence this. *NVQ/SVQ Focus and Care Standard*. Vol. 2, No. 9, pp40–42.

Day, M. and Basford, L. (1995). Fit for care. *Nursing Times*. Vol. 91, No. 14, pp42–43.

Debling, G. (1989). The Employment Department/Training Agency standards programme and National Vocational Qualifications: Implications for education. In Burke, J.W. (Ed.) *Competency-based Education and Training*. London: Falmer Press.

Dickson, N. and Cole, A. (1987). Nurse's little helper? *Nursing Times*. Vol. 83, No. 10, pp24–26.

Elliot, J. (1991). *Action Research for Educational Change*. Milton Keynes: Open University Press.

Employment Department (1988). *Employment for the 1990s*. Cm.540. London: HMSO.

Fletcher, S. (1991). *Designing Competence-Based Training*. London: Kogan Page.

Further Education Unit (1986). *Assessment, Quality and Competence: Staff Training issues for NCVQ*. London: F.E.U.

Further Education Unit (1987). *Competency-Based Vocational Education. FEU/PICKUP Project Report*. Dorset: Blackmore Press.

Further Education Unit (1989). *Implications of Competence-based Curricula*. London: F.E.U.

Giles, C. (1993). Assessors and verifiers – questions of qualification. *The NVQ Monitor*. Autumn Edition. London: NCVQ, p3.

Greenacre, L. (1990). Competence and coherence: opportunities for Education and Industry in the emerging National Vocational Qualifications framework. In Bees, M. and Swords, M. (Eds.) *National Vocational Qualifications and Further Education*. London: Kogan Page and NCVQ.

Hardie, M. (1987). A special kind of person. *Nursing Times*. Vol. 83, No. 10, pp26,27.

Jessup, G. (1991). *Outcomes: NVQs and the Emerging Model of Education and Training.* London: Falmer Press.

Joint Awarding Bodies (1992). *National Vocational Qualifications in Care: Notes on Assessment and Verification.* London: J.A.B

Lawton, D. (1973). *Social Change, Educational Theory and Curriculum Planning.* London: Hodder and Stoughton.

Manpower Services Commission (1981). *A New Training Initiative. Agenda for Action.* London: HMSO.

Manpower Services Commission (1986). *Review of Vocational Qualifications in England and Wales.* London: HMSO.

Mathias, P. (1993). Assessment requirements, knowledge and the log sheet. *Care Standard.* Vol. 1, No. 6, pp6,7.

McCrory, R. (1992). *Understanding National Vocational Qualifications and Standards: A handbook.* Lancs: Parthenon.

McMurray, A. (1986). Preceptoring. *Australia Nurses Journal.* Vol. 16, No. 3, pp43,44

Mitchell, L. (1993). NVQs/SVQs at higher levels: a discussion paper to the 'Higher Levels' Seminar, October 1992. *Competence and Assessment Briefing Series.* No. 8. Sheffield: Employment Department.

Mullin, R. (1992). *Decisions and Judgements in NVQ-based assessment. Report 14.* London: National Council for Vocational Qualifications.

National Council for Vocational Qualifications (1989). *National Vocational Qualifications: Criteria and Procedures.* London: NCVQ.

National Council for Vocational Qualifications (1990). *Accreditation of Prior Learning in the context of National Vocational Qualifications. Research and Development Report No. 7.* London: NCVQ.

National Council Vocational Qualifications (1992a). *Brief Guide NVQs and Work.* London: NCVQ.

National Council Vocational Qualifications (1992b). *NVQ Notes Assessing Competence in unpaid Work.* London: NCVQ.

National Council Vocational Qualifications (1992c). *NVQ Notes Access and Equal Opportunities.* London: NCVQ.

National Council Vocational Qualifications (1992d). *Brief Guide NVQs and Employers.* London: NCVQ.

National Council for Vocational Qualifications (1993). The Awarding Bodies Common Accord. London: NCVQ.

National Council for Vocational Qualifications (1995). *NVQ Criteria and Guidance.* London: NCVQ.

National Foundation for Educational Research (1991). *The NFER*

Project 2000 Research. The Experience of Planning and Initial Implementation. [Interim Paper No. 3.] Slough: NFER.

National Health Service Training Directorate (1991). *Occupational Standards for NVQ Assessors Training Resource Pack.* Bristol: NHSTD.

Nursing Times (1989). View from the frontline. *Nursing Times.* Vol. 85, No. 7, pp32,33.

Robertson, D. (1991). Courses, qualifications and the empowerment of learners. In Finegold, D., et al. (1991) *Higher Education Expansion and Reform.* Institute for Public Policy Research.

Royal Society of Arts (1991). *Accreditation of Prior Achievement.* Coventry: Royal Society of Arts Examination Board.

Simosko, S. (1991). *Accreditation of Prior Learning: A practical guide for professionals.* London: Kogan Page.

Stenhouse, L. (1975). *An Introduction to Curriculum Research and Development.* London: Heinemann.

Storey, L. (1991). Points of view. *Nursing Standard.* Vol. 5, No. 24, p43.

Storey, L., O'Kell, S. and Day, M. (1995). *Utilising National Occupational Standards as a Complement to Nursing Curricula.* Leeds: NHS Executive.

Trades Union Congress (1989). *Skills 2000.* London: TUC.

Training and Development Lead Body (1992). *National Standards for Training and Development.* Sheffield, Moorfoot: Employment Department.

Training and Development Lead Body (1995). *National Standards for Training and Development.* Sheffield, Moorfoot: Employment Department.

United Kingdom Central Council for Nursing and Midwifery (1986). *Project 2000: A new preparation for practice.* London: UKCC.

Waxman, L. (1993). A look at centre approval, quality and the D Units. *Care Standard.* Vol. 1, No. 10, p8.

Whitear, G. (1993). *The NVQ Handbook: A guide to career success.* London: Pitman.

Williams, K. (1989). *Study Skills.* London: Macmillan.

Glossary

Accredited Centre	An organisation that has been approved by an Awarding Body to deliver NVQs.
Assessment Record	Issued by the Awarding Body. When completed by the candidate and assessor it is a log of competence achieved.
APL	Accreditation of Prior Learning and Achievement.
Assessment	The process of judging a person's competence based upon the evidence presented.
Assessor	Someone licensed by an Accredited Centre to assess candidates for their NVQ Award. This person should be occupationally competent and hold TDLB units D32 and (or) D33.
BTEC	Business and Technology Education Council, an NVQ Awarding Body.
Candidate	Someone who is registered for an NVQ award.
Care Sector Consortium	The Lead Body and Occupational Standards Council for Care. Responsible for developing occupational standards in care.
CCETSW	Central Council for the Education and Training in Social Work, an NVQ Awarding Body.
Certification	Certificate issued by an Awarding Body in recognition of Unit accreditation, or the achievement of a whole NVQ award.
Competence	The ability to perform to nationally agreed standards within the workplace.
Core Unit	See *Unit*.
Credit accumulation	The process by which a candidate is credited for units that make up a complete NVQ award.

Element	An element outlines the specific activities which make up a unit of competence.
Endorsement Unit	See *Unit*.
External Verifier	See *Verification*.
Internal Verifier	See *Verification*.
JAB	Joint Awarding Bodies for NVQs in Care, including CCETSW and City and Guilds.
LEC	Local Enterprise Company. The local body responsible for instigating, monitoring and supporting training initiatives in Scotland. It provides a source of information and possible funding for NVQ candidates.
Level	Term used to describe degrees of competence which are based on the complexity and responsibility attached to an individual's occupation.
NCVQ	National Council for Vocational Qualifications.
NVQ	National Vocational Qualification, an award which is accredited by NCVQ.
NVQ Framework	A national system which places NVQs into appropriate occupational areas and levels of competence.
Performance Criteria	The standard of performance expected of a candidate.
Portfolio	A collection of material which is presented to the assessor as evidence of achievement.
Range	A statement describing the breadth and context in which the performance criteria must be achieved.
SCOTVEC	Scottish Council for Vocational Qualifications.
SVQ	Scottish Vocational Qualification, the equivalent of an NVQ.
TDLB	Training and Development Lead Body, who have devised NVQ units for Assessors (D32 and D33), Internal Verifiers (D33 and D34) and External Verifiers (D35).
TEC	Training and Enterprise Council. The local body responsible for instigating, monitoring and supporting training initiatives in Eng-

land and Wales. It provides a source of information and possible funding for NVQ candidates.

Testimonial | An account written by an employer or professional colleague which substantiates a candidate's claim to competence.

Underpinning knowledge | The knowledge required to support performance.

Unit | The smallest part of an NVQ award that is certificated.

Core Unit | A unit which is the basic building block of an NVQ in Care award, e.g. *U4. Contribute to the health, safety and security of individuals and their environment.* There are 6 Core Units at Level 2, and 8 Core Units at Level 3.

Endorsement Unit | Unit of competence that is specific to an occupational area of health care delivery, e.g. *Unit Z10 Enable clients to eat and drink* is one of the *Direct Care* Endorsement Units.

'O' Unit | The *'O' Unit* or Value Base is a Core Unit that describes the moral and ethical standards required of the health care worker. It covers effective communication, confidentiality, anti-discrimination, rights and choice, beliefs and identity. It is assessed throughout all of the units composing an NVQ in Care Award.

Verification | The process by which NVQ assessors are monitored and evaluated.

External Verifier | Appointed by the awarding body to monitor and evaluate the Accredited Centre. Holds TDLB Unit D35.

Internal Verifier | Someone licensed by the Accredited Centre to monitor, evaluate and develop the work of NVQ assessors. Normally an experienced assessor who holds TDLB units D33 and D34.